Enrich Your Life

World's Classics

100 Greatest Novels of All Time

www.iboo.com

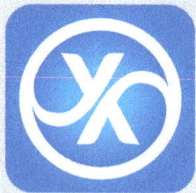

I'M ON THE SAME PAGE

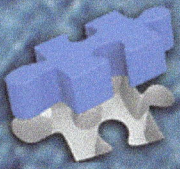

CREATIVE EDGE PUBLICITY

Your brand. Your future.

+1 403-464-6925
www.creative-edge.services

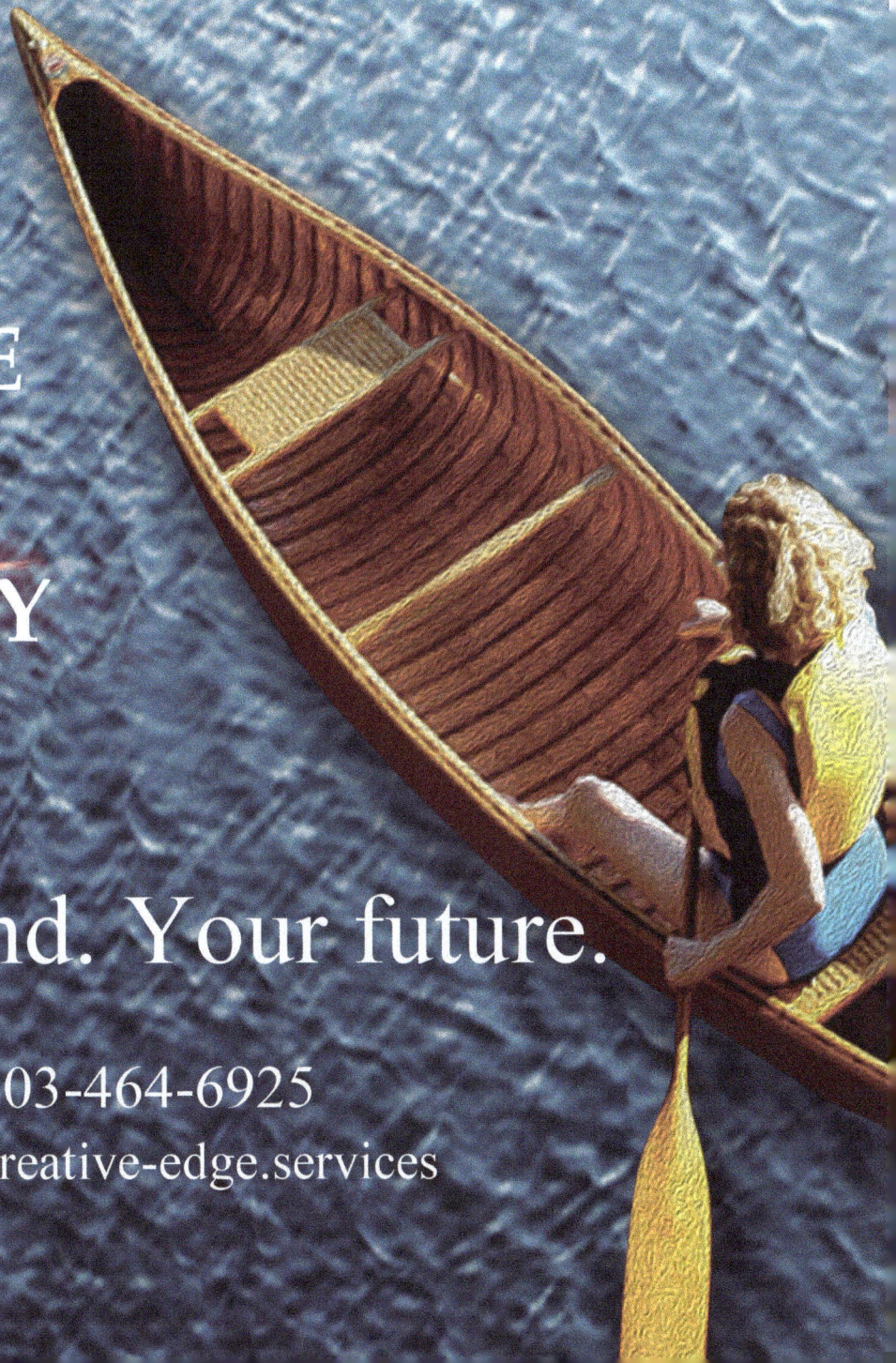

Save
The Ocean

Feed
The World

OCEANA

Restoring the oceans could feed 1 billion people a healty seafood meal each day

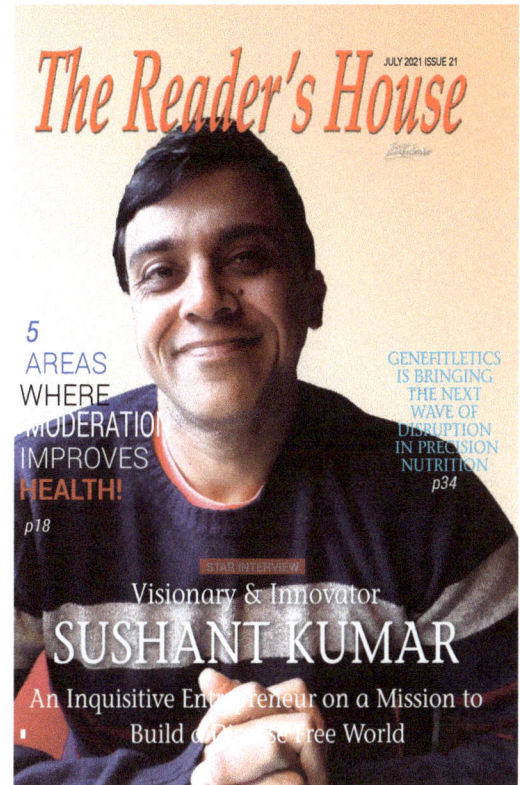

JULY 2021 ISSUE 21

The Reader's House

5 AREAS WHERE MODERATION IMPROVES HEALTH! p18

GENEFITLETICS IS BRINGING THE NEXT WAVE OF DISRUPTION IN PRECISION NUTRITION p34

STAR INTERVIEW

Visionary & Innovator
SUSHANT KUMAR

An Inquisitive Entrepreneur on a Mission to Build a Disease Free World

In this Issue

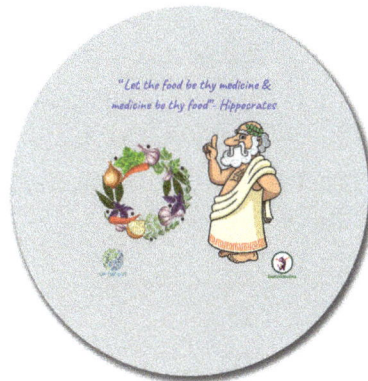

"Let the food be thy medicine & medicine be thy food"- Hippocrates

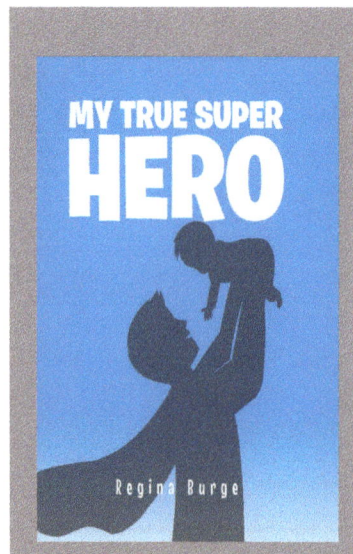

In this Issue

MY TRUE SUPER HERO

Regina Burge

EDITOR'S LETTER

We're so proud to connect writers, authors, artists, coaches, doctors who are always ready to share their story and passion with an interview, and we put them to The Reader's House spotlight.

On our cover is *Sushant Kumar* is a visionary entrepreneur, innovator, who believes that a curious & inquisitive mindset is what will drive a person to create value for others. Having held leadership positions for 2 decades across diverse sectors & built businesses in healthcare & financial services, coupled with his own transformation struggle from obese nerd to a healthy soul, puts him in a unique position to embark on a journey to help people improve their health.

We continue to connect people. We have interviewed not just acclaimed, as well as award winning authors like *Jennifer Anne Gordon*, a gothic horror/literary fiction novelist, won the Kindle Award for Best Horror/Suspense for 2020, Won Best Horror 2020 from Authors on the Air, was a Finalist for American Book Fest's Best Book Award- Horror, 2020. She also received the Platinum 5 Star Review from Reader's Choice as well as the Gold Seal from Book View.

We featured Enlightened Thought Leader *Dr. Chérie Carter-Scott* on the cover of March issue. *Dr Chérie* is #1 New York Times Best Selling Author (19 Books), Oprah Winfrey Endorsed, Consultant to Fortune 500 companies.

International Bestselling Author *Kathrin Hutson*, NY Times Bestseller Author *Tosca Lee*, Acclaimed crime fiction Canadian Author, *Melissa Yi*, Past President of the Sisters In Crime NJ and Award Winning Author, **Kristina Rienzi** are some of authors we will feature on the cover in upcoming issues.

Enjoy Reading

A. Harlowe

The Reader's House

Published by Newyox

LONDON OFFICE
3rd Floor
86-90 Paul Street
London
EC2A 4NE UK

t: +44 20 3828 7097
editor@newyox.com
newyox.com

Editor in Chief
Anna Harlow
Managing Director
Dan Peters
Marketing Director
Ben Alan

CONTRIBUTORS

Mickey Mikkelson
Rian Donatelli
George Uliano
Nick Wehrli
Andy Machin
By Hakeem Hashmi Amroha-Hashmi
Dawakhana
Lisa Brown Gilbert

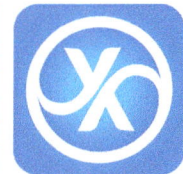

Visionary & Innovator
SUSHANT KUMAR
An Inquisitive Entrepreneur on a Mission to Build a Disease Free World

"Attitude, competence & execution are three core pillars to conquer this world & bring positive differences in the lives of people. If you have these three, the sky's the limit for you."

BY DAN PETERS
MAY 21, 2021

Tell us about yourself and your company. What kind of Corporation is your business?

I'm a visionary entrepreneur, innovator, inventor who believes that a curious & inquisitive mindset is what will drive a person to create value for others. Having held leadership positions for 2 decades across diverse sectors & built businesses in healthcare & financial services, coupled with my own transformation struggle from obese nerd to a healthy soul, puts me in a unique position to embark on a journey to help people improve their health. "Attitude, competence & execution are three core pillars to conquer this world & bring positive differences in the lives of people. If you have these three, the sky's the limit for you." I'm on a mission to build a disease free world by shaking hands with invisible forces at work inside our body- genes & gut microbes.

My company Genefitletics, is an evidence based biotech solution that sequences human & gut microbiome DNA to decode health insights and biomarkers of more than 30 chronic diseases & analyse the interaction between food & gut microbes through saliva & stool samples to provide a personalised nutrition solution.

What is the problem you are solving & what is unique about your business?

52% of the global adult population is suffering from chronic diseases due to imbalance in gut bacteria, leaky gut & disturbed circadian rhythm resulting in chronic diseases. Given the fact that 41 million meet premature death globally, our current disease based model of medicine has been ineffective in dealing with chronic diseases.

The key stakeholders of the healthcare sector- doctors, hospitals & insurance companies do not make money until the patient remains sick & requires constant consulting & medication. These solutions which place antibiotics & surgeries over curing the patients, do long term collateral damage & have a cascading impact on overall health, thereby driving people towards life threatening disorders.

Our business replaces this current model with a human biology based

Continued *on page 16*

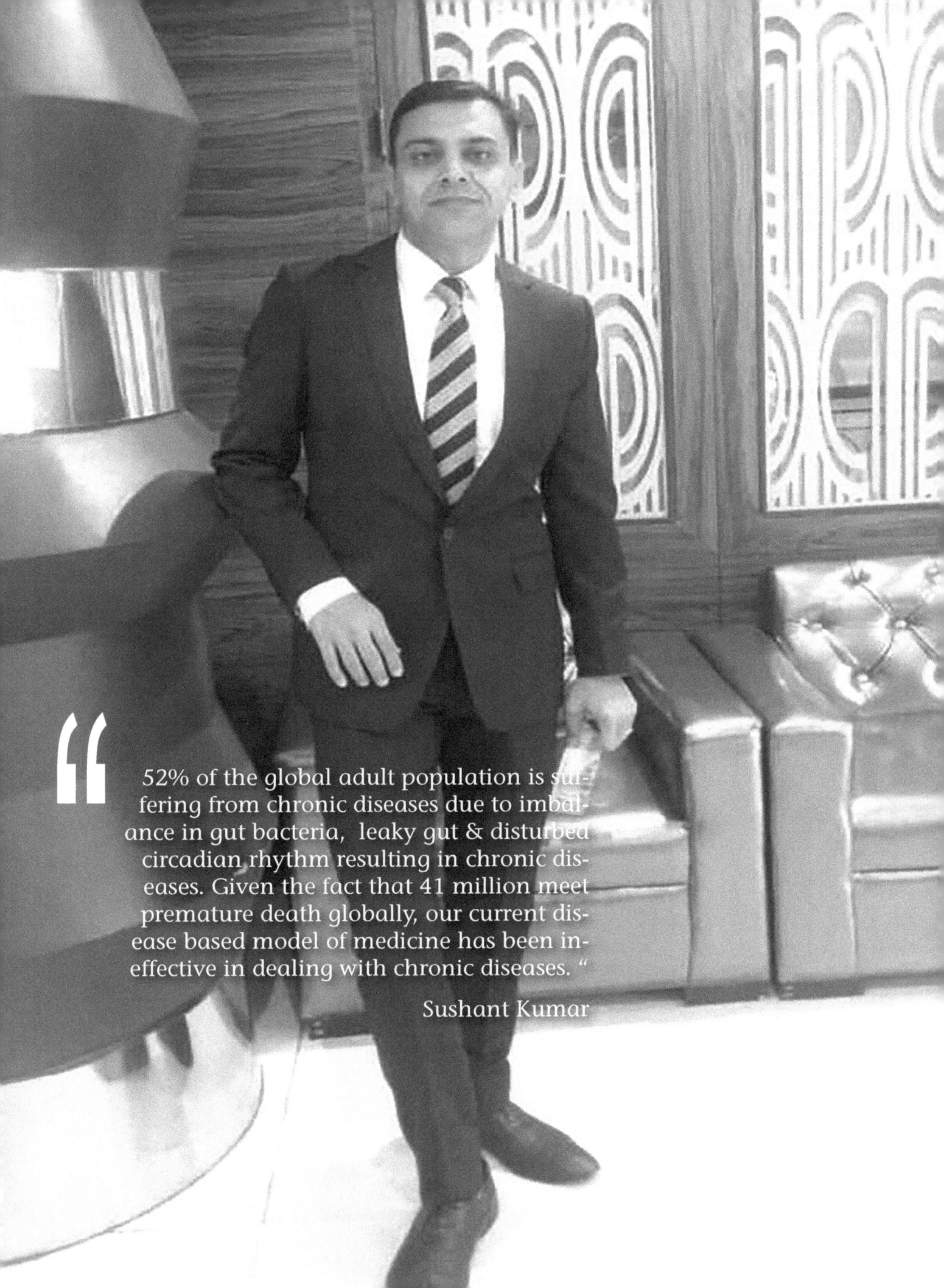

> "52% of the global adult population is suffering from chronic diseases due to imbalance in gut bacteria, leaky gut & disturbed circadian rhythm resulting in chronic diseases. Given the fact that 41 million meet premature death globally, our current disease based model of medicine has been ineffective in dealing with chronic diseases. "
>
> Sushant Kumar

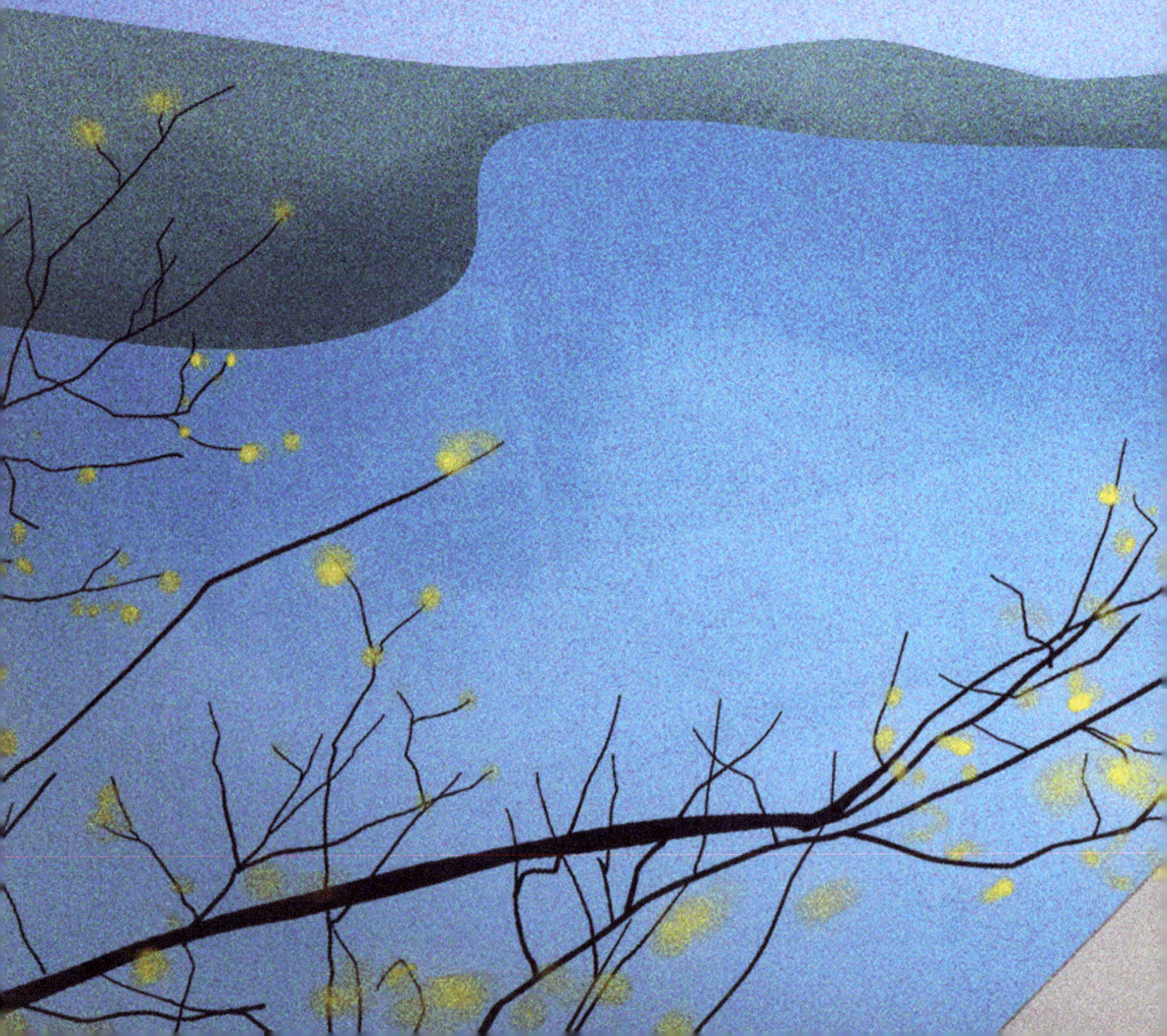

It's time to take a stand for homeless pets. It's time to adopt change. Every day, more than 4,100 dogs and cats are killed in shelters across the country — but **with Best Friends Animal Society leading the way, and your support, we can help our nation's shelters and Save Them All**

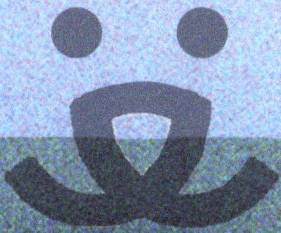

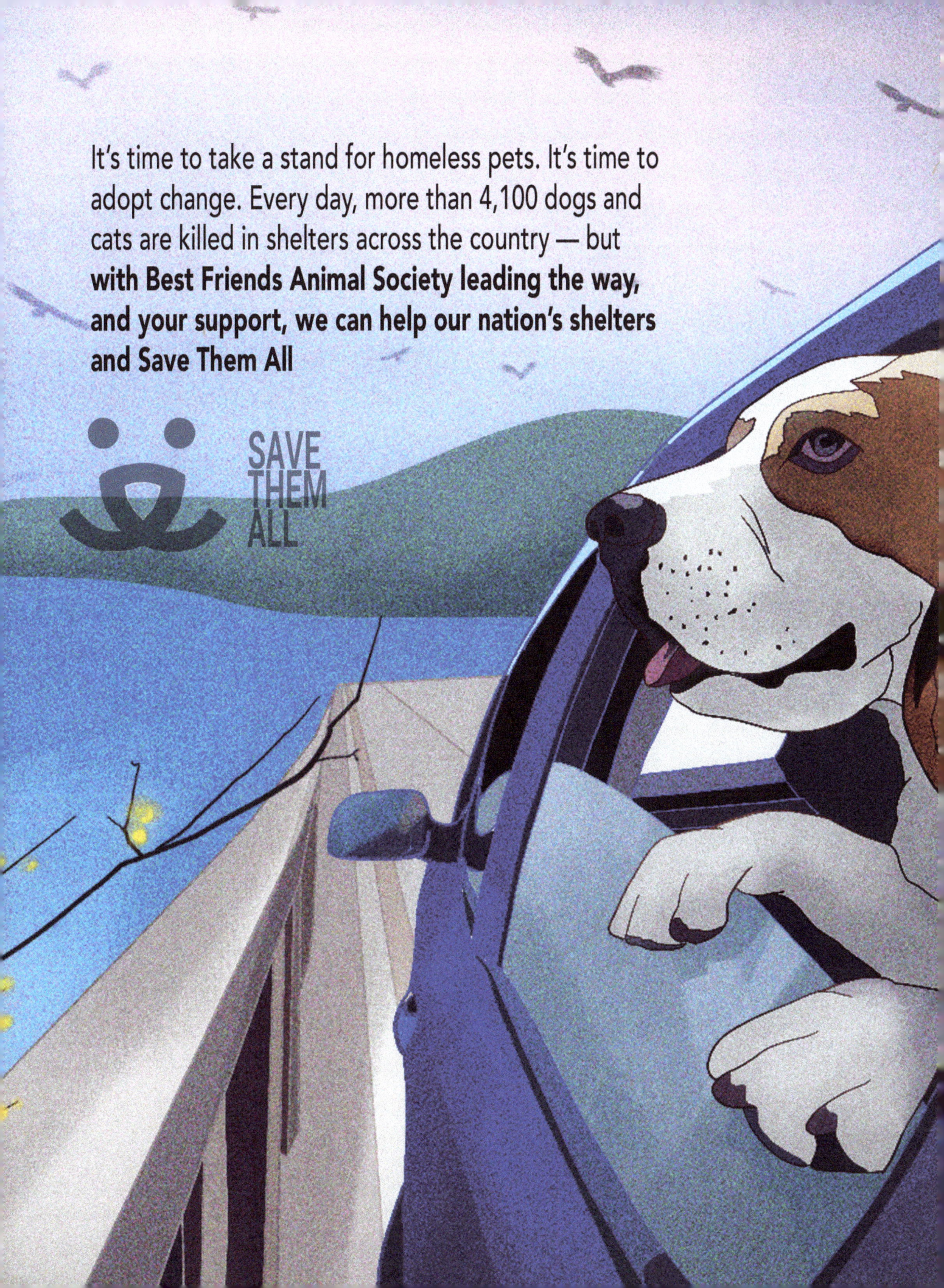

SAVE
THEM
ALL

COVID-19
What Should I Do?

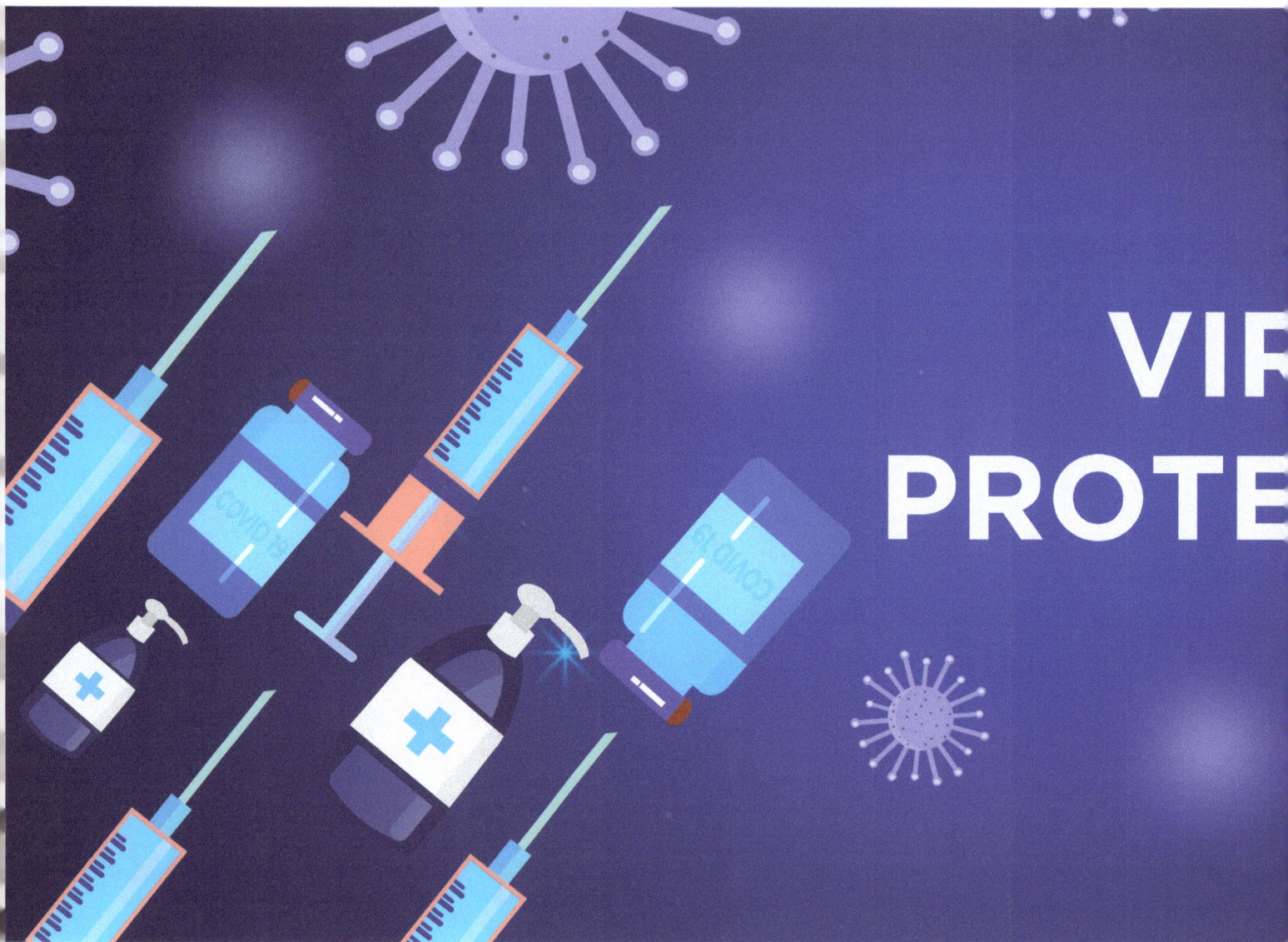

VIR
PROTE

Think of it this way over 95% of every American as been vaccinated against Polio, measles, mumps, and other child-hood diseases. How many Children and Babies would have died if their parents refused to get them vaccinated.

BY GEORGE ULIANO

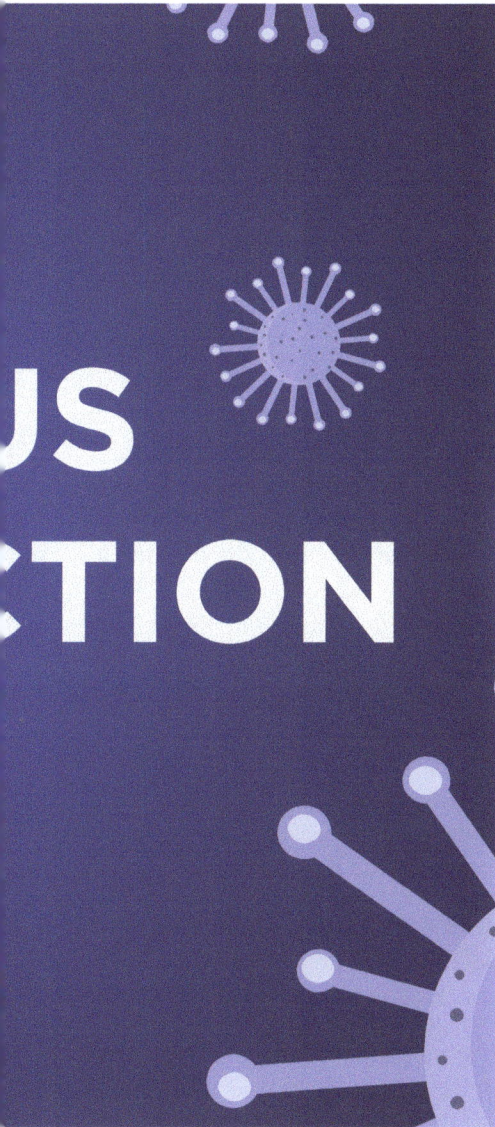

It has been over a year since the Covid19 Pandemic struck the world. What should you do now? First, I am not a Doctor, I do not even have a background in the medical field. My background is in the security and lock business. I do have a lot of common sense and I can separate the hype from reality.

Unfortunately, it was an election year when this virus hit. That made it political. Both parties should be ashamed of themselves. I honestly believe that if politics were not involved less people would have died. Decisions were made based on politics not what was the best for the American people. That continues today.

The news outlets have also turned political. I remember a time that when you tuned into the news you felt that you were getting the truth with no bias. Today that is also very different, and that difference has also cost American lives. The news media is very quick to report anything without doing their own research. This causes them to give the wrong information to people, again costing lives.

Fortunately, people have caught on to this and now get their news form multiple sources that they trust. Therefore, newspapers are closing down, and people are "cutting the cord" going to what they want to watch by streaming.

So, what should you do Now? Well, it seems that infections, hospitalization, and deaths are going down. The consensus from the Medical Experts is that by fall we should be back to normal, whatever that is. You should do what seems right to you. Use your common sense. Get your news from as many different sources as you can.

In my opinion everyone should get the vaccine. I realize that there has been some resistance from some people. I think that this resistance is age related. Older people over 60 were quick to get the vaccine when offered, after all they were the age group that was dying. The younger generations not so much.

Think of it this way over 95% of every American as been vaccinated against Polio, measles, mumps, and other childhood diseases. How many Children and Babies would have died if their parents refused to get them vaccinated.

As adults getting a vaccine is your choice, do your research, make sure you research multiple reputable sources. Look for sources that DO NOT agree with your position, so you can get a clear picture of the other side. Then make the decision that is best for you.

George Uliano is a security professional with years of law enforcement and security experience. He earned a Bachelors Degree in Criminal Justice and Business graduating with honors. George holds three U.S. patents on different locking principles. This combination gives George and His Company Locking Systems International Inc the unique ability to provide its customers with the correct security at an affordable price.

For additional information or to purchase Locks go to http://www.lsidepot.com

Continued *from page 10*

model to understand how our body really works, how to run it optimally & fix the issues safely when something goes wrong.

Genefitletics offers unparalleled visibility into a human body to create a unique profile of biochemistry & microbial community & make personalised adaptable & actionable precision nutrition recommendations for improving the health of its customers.

Genefitletics is not just a genetic sequencing test, but the true health mascot for its customers. Our recommendations are adapted to your changing microbial profile & examine it regularly, so as to empower you to improve your healthspan & buoyancy.

This deep understanding of genes & gut living inside our body allows us to recommend to each individual as to why they should eat certain foods, and why they should avoid certain foods based on their own individual biology, with the goal to prevent and reverse chronic disease.

How and why did you get started in this line of work?

I was born and brought up in a traditional & stereotypical environment, where you are tutored to play safe throughout your life, secure a job and lead a simple blissful life. I used to be a typical finance professional in a secured job environment, so my life was all about travelling to & fro from my home to office. I was never satisfied or happy with this mediocre job mindset and running after money in a rat race. Things took an upside turn, when I went to pursue MBA from IE Business School, Spain. After meeting folks from every corner of the world,

I discovered that people are plagued with irrational and outdated healthcare practices, which were not helping them improve their health span. So I asked myself, "Can we envision a world which does not have any space for chronic ailments?"

I left with this thought when I came back from Spain. After witnessing a series of deaths of my loved ones in the family, and how others around them are impacted, I decided to build something that can help people become

> *"To be frank, I never felt under stress during the pandemic! All I did was follow precautions & guidelines issued by the government & maintained a healthy immunity. I made sure that I spent 2 hours every day on my workout which boosted & energy level. Besides, speaking with various people daily & listening & solving their health problems give me enough motivation & boost to keep going. "*

independent of any doctors & medicines & improve their healthspan.

That same time, I was diagnosed with fatty liver stage 3 and I was obese and weighed 105 Kgs. I had to transform myself first, for making my vision a reality & helping people.

While through a strong motivation & following a standard calorie deficit diet & regular workout I was able to transform myself from an obese man to a healthy soul, my overall health took a backseat & a huge toll on my gut. This made me realise the real problem in the healthcare delivery model- it is not focussed on curing people.

I was strongly opposed to this current model of healthcare where doctors, hospitals & insurance companies do not make money until the patient remains sick & requires constant consulting & medication. Truly, the pharmacy companies are the biggest wealth makers, because whatever they're manufacturing in their labs is not supposed to reverse the chronic diseases, it's just helping people manage their disease symptoms. It is more like delaying the effects of a disease.

I was inclined to fix the current healthcare model with the objective of mani-

festing & building a disease free world. I wanted to figure out what it takes to actually reverse these human diseases. Not having a typical healthcare background was never my concern. I research a lot of medical journals & scientific papers & all pointed out one common root cause of human diseases: the invisible army inside our gut- "the gut microbiome". We humans have only 25,000 genes , so how come the human body is such a complex system?

This led to a miraculous conclusion & believe that we humans have assigned the task of managing our health to trillions of microorganisms living in our gut having the number of genes almost 10^4 times those of humans. This further led to belief that it is these microbes who are decision makers in every aspect of human health. By optimising these microbiomes, humans can actually take care of their health without depending too much on medications.

Genefitletics was born with the objective of building a disease free world by sequencing human & gut microbiome DNA to decode health insights and biomarkers of more than 30 chronic diseases & analyze the interaction between food & gut microbes to provide personalised nutrition.

How do you deal with the stress of Covid-19?

To be frank, I never felt under stress during the pandemic! All I did was follow precautions & guidelines issued by the government & maintained a healthy immunity. I made sure that I spent 2 hours every day on my workout which boosted & energy level. Besides, speaking with various people daily & listening & solving their health problems give me enough motivation & boost to keep going.

What is most important to you in a

company?

Our business revolves around 3 pillars- customer, customer & customer. Solving customers' health problems & empowering them to improve their health span is the epicenter of our business.

What was the best part of business since the covid-19 started?

COVID-19 has led us to rethink & pivot our business model & build in

& neurodegenerative pathways to provide personalised dietary recommendations.

How does an individual benefit from your services?

Using functional analysis of human & gut microbial DNA, Genefitletics recommends a personalised diet for an individual along with unique recommendations which will,
•Focus on plant-based nutrition with personalised serving recommendations

dynamic science associated with human biology & overall health. We have been following this approach & engaging our users through our content & community building initiatives. One can find our blogs, articles, podcasts, webinars on www.genefitletics.com and become a member for free. We also engage our community by organising virtual events & challenges to help them with small tweaks in their lifestyle which definitely leads to development of healthy habits.

"Our business revolves around 3 pillars- customer, customer & customer. Solving customers' health problems & empowering them to improve their health span is the epicenter of our business."

To what do you attribute your success?

My passion & innate responsibility to bring positive impact in the lives of people

What's your company's goals?

To build a disease free world.

additional offerings that can help people alleviate their health issues. It has also driven people's attention towards their health. As a result, they are now looking for something beyond medicines to cure them effectively.

How covid-19 affected the way of doing business?

Covid-19 made us location independent & give access to multitude of resources & recruit people from different parts of the world.

What service(s) or product(s) do you offer/manufacture?

Genefitletics is currently offering two solutions:
1.Curegenic- This is a comprehensive biointelligence solution that analyses customers' genes & microbiomes through saliva & stool samples covering Metabolic health, Disease risk estimation, Genetic predisposition to intolerances & allergies, Inflammatory activity, Predisposition to drug addiction, Digestive efficiency, Microbiome profile & Circadian Rhythm to provide personalised dietary recommendations
2.UP THE GUT- This product analyses customer's microbiomes through stool samples covering metabolic, digestive

of animal and plant proteins and fats.
•Identify foods that are most aligned with his microbiome.
•Recommend a diet that will increase his energy and well being.
•Recommend a diet to help him achieve and maintain a healthy weight.

Do you work locally or nationally?

We work internationally, currently serving in India, Australia, Europe & Middle East.

Where do you see yourself in five years?

COVID-19 has led us to rethink & pivot our business model & build in additional offerings that can help people alleviate their health issues. It has also driven people's attention towards their health. As a result, they are now looking for something beyond medicines to cure them effectively.

In the

•Optimise his digestion and nutrient absorption.
•Optimise beneficial bacteria with probiotics.
End result: One can fine tune the function of his gut microbiome to minimise production of harmful metabolites & maximise production of beneficial ones, so that he can improve his energy levels, fine tune the immunity & prevent occurrence of chronic inflammation.

How do you advertise your business?

We do not believe that the healthcare business needs any advertisement. What the healthcare sector requires is, educating & information about

next 5 years I see myself as a healthcare entrepreneur, who has brought a positive impact in the lives of at least 200,000 people by improving their health condition.

If you had one piece of advice to someone just starting out, what would it be?

Just focus on the customer's problem and how you can make the customer's life better. ●

5 Areas Where Moderation Improves Health!

BY RICHARD BRODY

If, you have eaten, a certain way/ diet, etc, for many years, changing, dramatically, overnight, may seem, overwhelming, and, thus, this becomes, one of the key reasons, so many diets, and weight - loss plans, fail!

Photos by Nick Wehrli

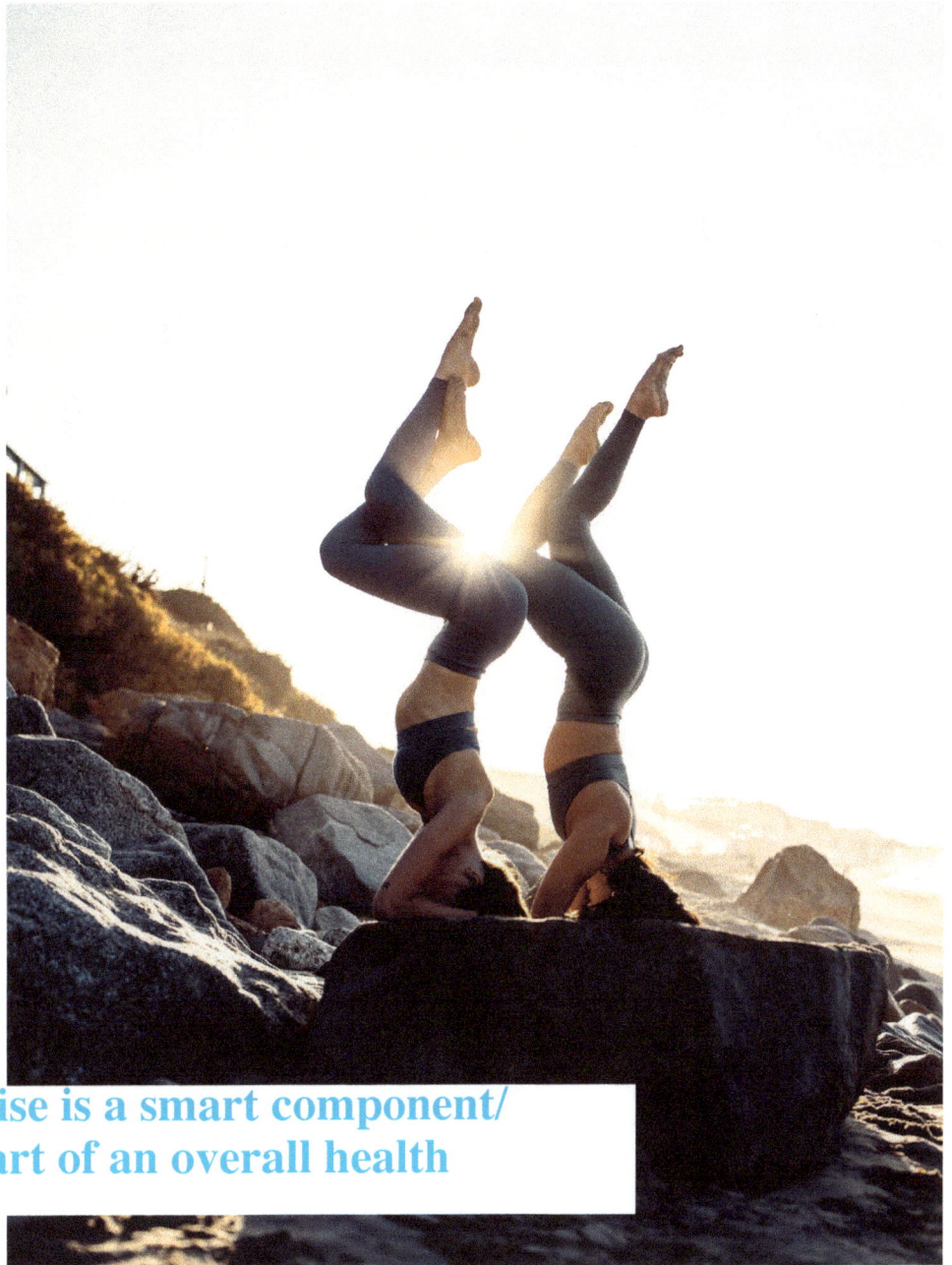

exercise is a smart component/ part of an overall health

When, it comes to, our health, and well - being, it often takes, a considerable amount of discipline and commitment, to maximize our possibilities! One of the essential lessons, to learn, and heed, is, using moderation, in a variety of areas, where doing so, is possible, and may, make sense! Doesn't it, make sense, it may be easier, to pursue, our personal best - interests, if, instead of trying, to, over - do things/ actions/ behaviors, we proceeded, with ways, which seemed, more plausible, and made the transitions/ changes, appear, more reasonable, etc? With, that in mind, this article will attempt to, briefly, consider, examine, review, and discuss, 5 areas, where this, will often, improve our overall health, and well - being.

1. Eating habits: If, you have eaten, a certain way/ diet, etc, for many years, changing, dramatically, over-night, may seem, overwhelming, and, thus, this becomes, one of the key reasons, so many diets, and weight - loss plans, fail! A more - moderate, sensible approach, might be, pursu-ing, a step - by - step, baby step's, approach, and researching options, and alternatives, considering, your personal needs, and what foods, you most desire, and coming - up, with a viable, applicable, solution!

2. Drinking - in moderation: Unless, one has alcohol dependency, issues/ challenges, and, enjoys, having an occasional drink, drinking - in mod-eration, may be a sensible approach! Don't drink, because you feel, you

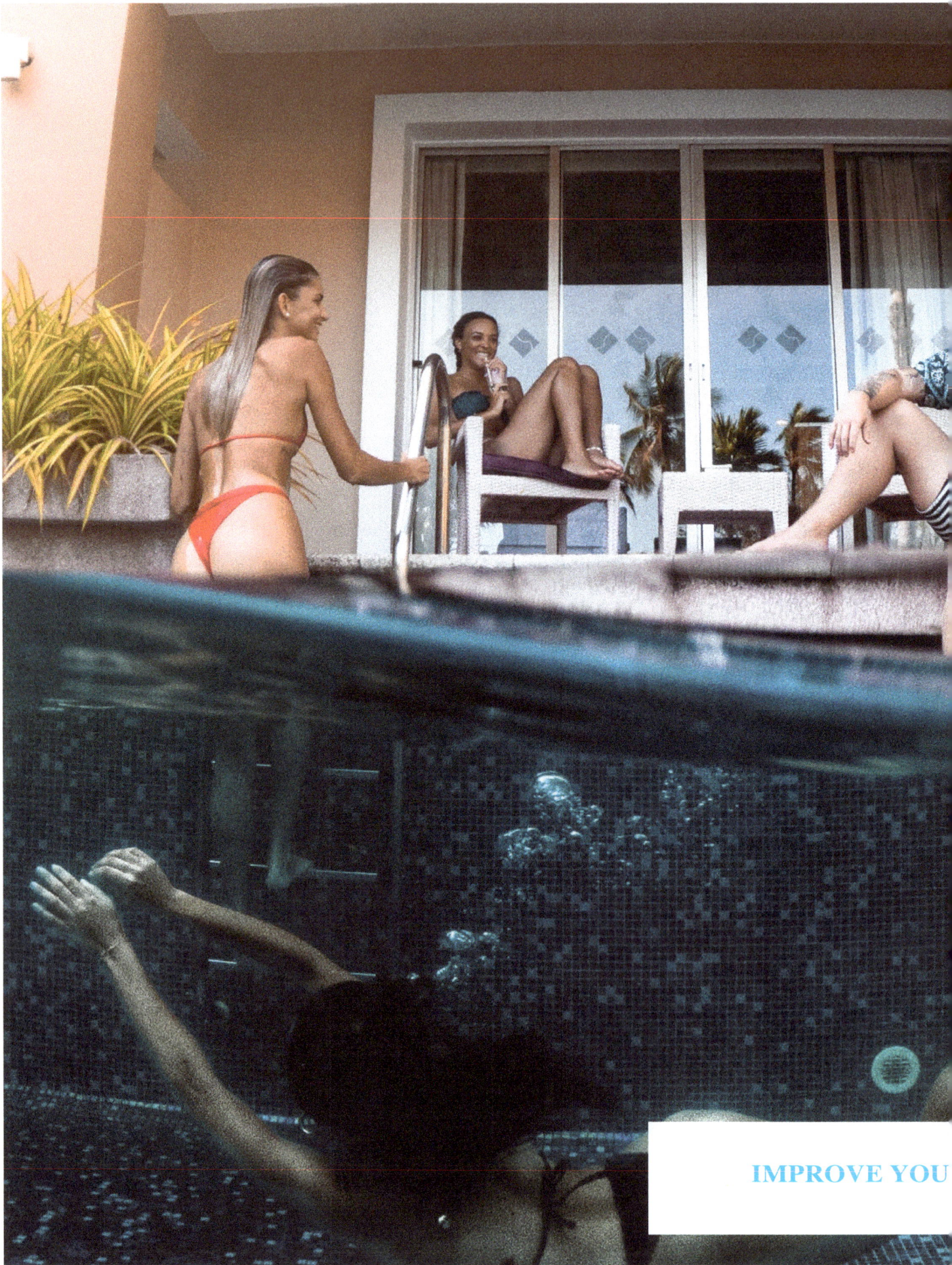

IMPROVE YOU

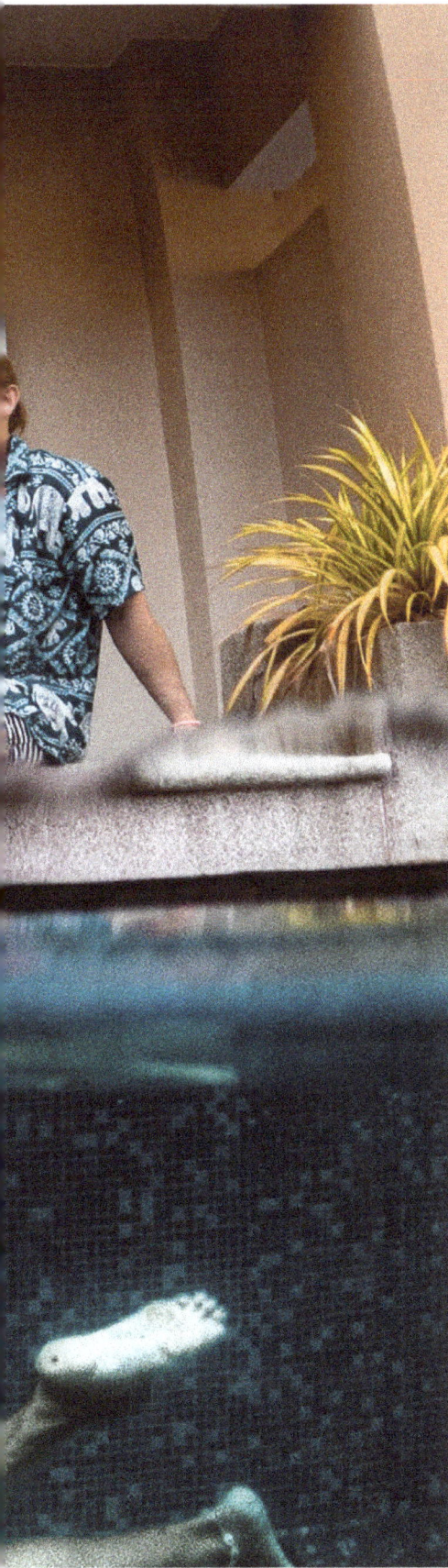

disipline
and comitment
are the rule

need one, but, rather, only, when you want one! Discover, what you enjoy, and why, and do so, occasionally, but, not, all the time! Never use drinking as a crutch, or excuse, for anti - social behavior!

3. Lifestyle - related: During our life, our needs, lifestyle, overall health, etc, may, often, change, several times! It is foolish to attempt to, live the same lifestyle, when you are 50, and over, as you did, when you were in your twenties, and thirties! Some of these areas, when moderating behaviors, may be personally, helpful, include, bed - time (amount of sleep, needed, etc), social activities, dinner - time, etc.

4. Exercise: Appropriate exercise, is, usually, a smart component/ part of an overall health, and well - being, program, and approach! One should consult his trusted, health professional, especially, when, either making significant changes, or embarking, on something new,

from an exercise - perspective!

5. Control temper/ anger: There may, at - times, be, a fine - line, between, controlling one's temper, and anger levels, and holding things - in, excessively! Finding a smart compromise, which works, for you, is beneficial, and worthwhile!

If you hope to enjoy a healthier, happier life, doesn't it make sense, to proceed, with well - considered, moderation? Will you be willing to give yourself, a much - needed, checkup - from - the - neck - up. to find, how to use, moderation, for your best, personal results?

Richard has owned businesses, been a COO, CEO, Director of Development, consultant, professionally run events, consulted to thousands, and conducted personal development seminars, for 4 decades. Rich has written three books and thousands of articles. His company, PLAN-2LEAD, LLC has an informative website http://plan2lead.net and Plan2lead can also be followed on Facebook http://facebook.com/Plan-2lead

ERALL HEALTH, AND WELL - BEING.

Regina Burge's New Book,

'My True Super Hero' Is A Brilliant Work That Gives A Beautiful Display Of Familial Love

Fulton Books author Regina Burge, a teacher, an active member of the church, and a mother of three wonderful sons, has completed her most recent book "My True Super Hero": a wonderful journal of a girl's memories shared with her father from her childhood to becoming a grown up.

GARFIELD HEIGHTS, Ohio, May 26, 2021 (Newswire.com) - Fulton Books author Regina Burge, a teacher, an active member of the church, and a mother of three wonderful sons, has completed her most recent book "My True Super Hero": a wonderful journal of a girl's memories shared with her father from her childhood to becoming a grown up.

Regina writes, "In a world full of adventure, children get to experience many great superheroes, but it's not often they get to show off the ones in their very own lives. This book will allow you the opportunity to use your bragging rights to applaud the superhero in your life—that person that works hard to change the world every day just for you. And that's what makes them a true superhero."

MY TRUE SUPER HERO

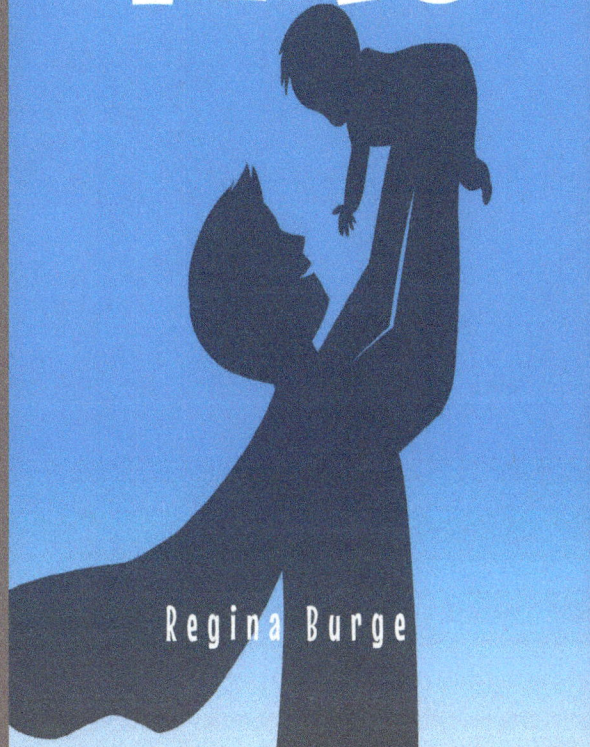

Regina Burge

Published by Fulton Books, Regina Burge's book is an admiring piece that lets readers recognize and honor their superheroes in life - may it be their own parents, grandparents, teachers, etc., and show gratitude to them. It also inspires the readers to be instruments of others by doing their obligations and living the values in the relationship that God desires.

Readers who wish to experience this great work can purchase "My True Super Hero" at bookstores everywhere, or online at the Apple iTunes store, Amazon, Google Play or Barnes and Noble.

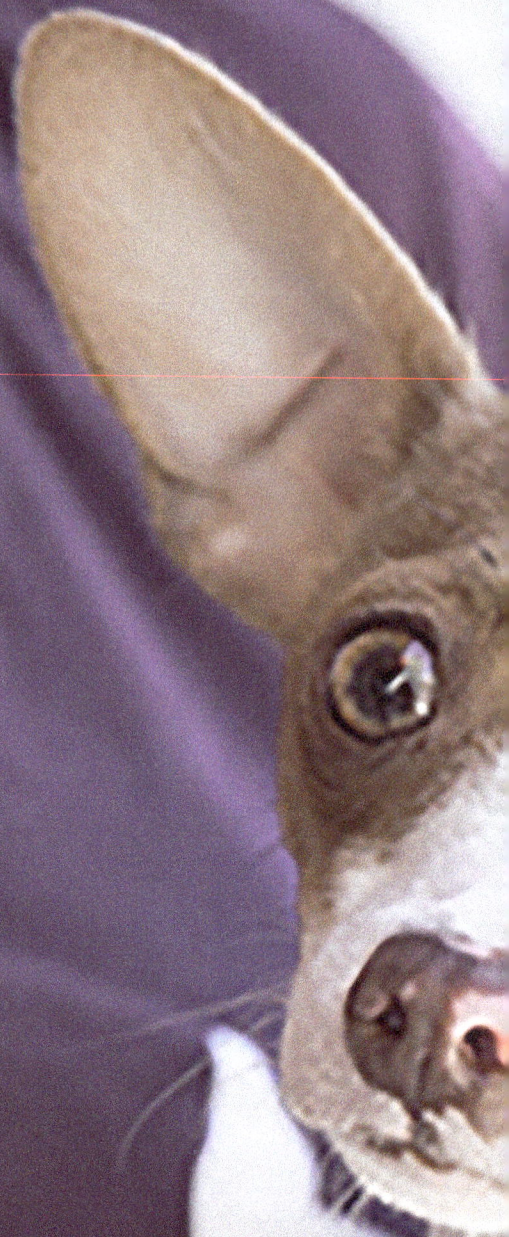

WE WILL NOT TAKE THIS SITTING DOWN

It's time to take a stand for homeless pets. It's time to adopt change. Every day, more than 4,100 dogs and cats are killed in shelters across the country — but **with Best Friends Animal Society leading the way, and your support, we can help our nation's shelters and Save Them All**

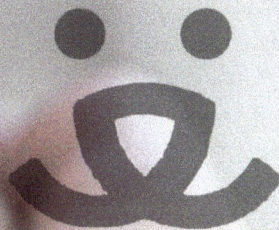

SAVE
THEM
ALL

IMPORTANCE OF
WEDDING NIGHT
IN LIFE

BY HAKEEM HASHMI
AMROHA-HASHMI
DAWAKHANA

> THE MOMENTS OF THE FIRST MEETING ARE VERY PRECIOUS MOMENTS IN LIFE. IF A MAN IS NOT ABLE TO HANDLE HIMSELF WITH HASTE ON HIS RUDE BEHAVIOR THEN UNFORTUNATELY HIS WEDDING NIGHT TURNS INTO NIGHT.

First contact on a wedding night is not limited to only physical contact, but also bounded to the mental and spiritual contact. It is believed that in this moment, two bodies become one life and leads to the golden future of a successful life. It is also said that its foundation should be very strong so that the ups and downs of time could not make relationship spoil. On the night of beginning of a relationship, couple needs to understand each other. Often, couple prefers to go somewhere outside after marriage like on mountainous place or on private place in solitude and have the curiosity to know each other deeply. Because it is very difficult for newlywed couple to understand each other at a house filled with relatives and other families who have come to the wedding. It is prevalent in all countries and is equally important everywhere.

If you are not able to become the true life partner of your new bride, then you will not be able to become a partner on the bed and your bride will start considering you as bad and lustful person and consider herself as scapegoat. Therefore, the moments of the first meeting are very precious moments in life. If a man is not able to handle himself with haste on his rude behavior then unfortunately his wedding night turns into night.

Today's, girls are also educated and understand the current scenario of the society well. Due to which every girl keeps a happy picture of her married life in her heart and wants her husband according to the same picture. If the husband is successful in winning the heart of his new bride, then it is definitely the beginning of his married life.

It is said that on the first night, the husband should never be rash for sexual intercourse rather he should praise every object like appearance, color, eyes, lips, nose, face texture and clothes etc. Do

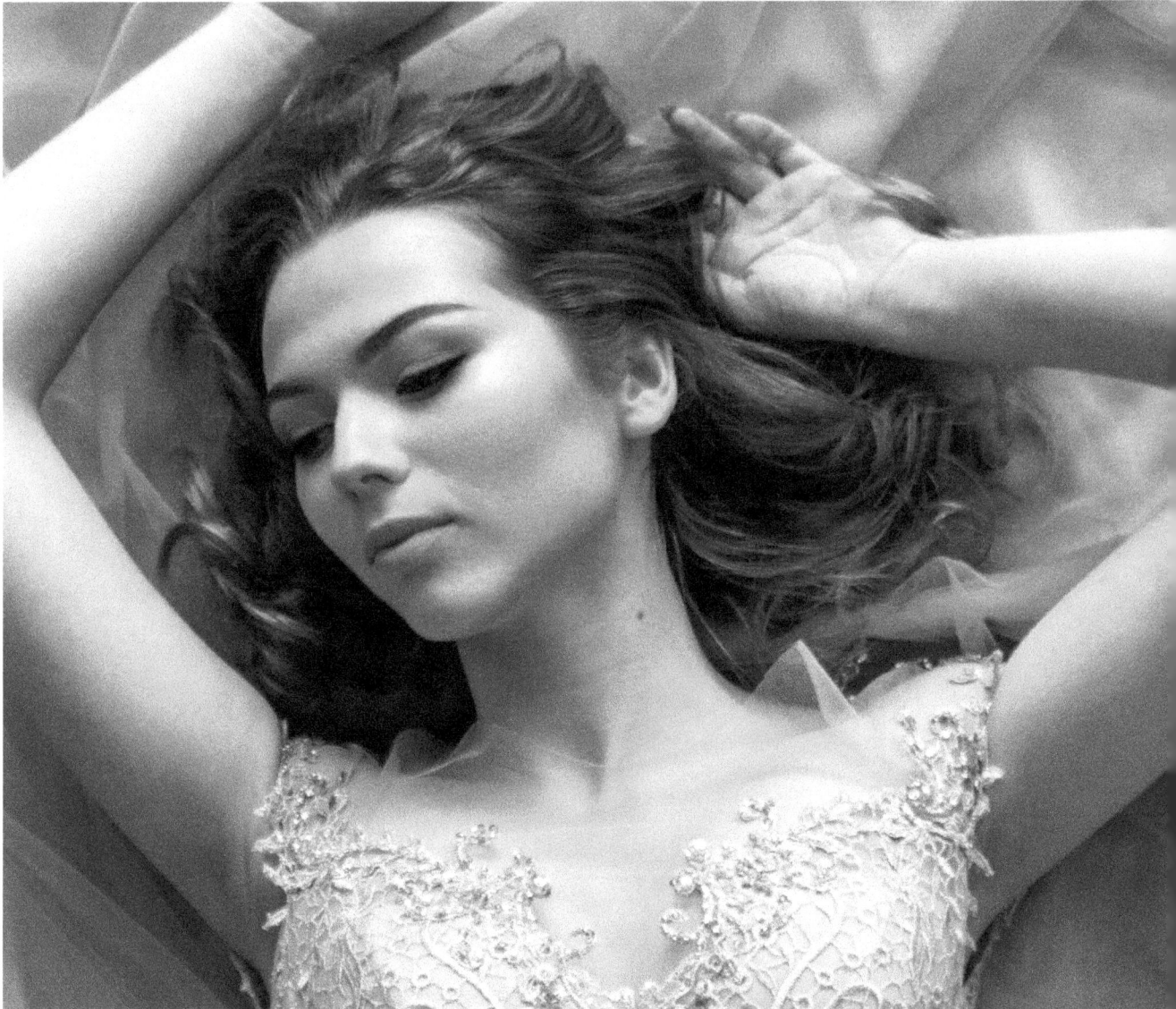

not praise the beauty and qualities of any other girl or woman in front of your new bride because it will affect your wife and she will not be able to give full support to you. First, subdue the mind of your wife and keep control over yourself to a limit. Once she will be enamored by you as a lover and successful man, she will surrender herself to you with happiness and full support. For the new bride, first time cohabitation is painful so first of all taking care of her sufferings and try to remove her hesitation slowly.

In my opinion, intake of alcohol or any drugs should not be consumed in wedding night else it might have a bad effect on their upcoming married life. This night comes only once in a life and women and men tie the memories of this night in a knot for the rest of their lives. Some ignorant people believe that it is necessary to have blood come on the first night from brides vaginal and it is a sign of bride's character. This is not true, their concepts are absolutely wrong. Because some girls have very tight vaginal membranes while others have very thin and soft membranes which may burst due to childhood injuries such as involving into sports, get up and down from buses and trains and through a rapid jerk etc. As a result of bursting of membranes before sex, there is no question of blood come from brides vaginal. So in absence of blood, do not doubt in vain on character of your new bride. Otherwise, married life will become a flame of sorrows and your whole life will be devastated.

Source: Articlesfactory

BOOK REVIEW

Harbor's Edge by Sanne Rothman

BY LISA BROWN GILBERT

Follow the F.B.I. Criminal Profiling rules. Dig up secrets on a Hawaiian island. Accept that sometimes only evil can push you to love. Harbor has lost too much already, yet finds herself in a race to uncover clues that unlock a strange mystery linked not only to her dad's murder but to an ancient legend that links us all. Author Sanne Rothman presents the 1st novel featuring The Untold Legend of the MO'O, a shape-shifting water lizard that steals your soul right before your eyes...unless the heart is stolen first.

Sanne Rothman's young adult thriller, Harbor's Edge, piques the curiosity while romancing the imagination, with a story that offers mystery, the supernatural, budding romance, and an intelligent 14-year-old heroine on a profoundly insightful journey to self-discovery. The story is set in beautiful Hawaii with which author Sanne Rothman does a wonderful job of detailing the beautiful environment. She brings forth both its timeless natural beauty as well as artfully presents intriguing aspects of Hawaiian life and culture especially with her incorporation of the lore of the dark and ancient sea monsters called The Mo'o, the legend, and mystery of which is initially contemplated by Harbor early on in the story. Initially, as the story unfolds, we meet Harbor, a young, resilient, intelligent teenager who finds her life shrouded in mystery and sadness. Having lost both her parents under mysterious circumstances, she fights with feelings of abandonment as she seeks to solve the mystery of what truly happened. She lost her F.B.I. agent father to a cold-blooded murderer and her mother, who disappeared without a trace, leaving her and her younger sister Fig in the care of their TuTu (grandmother). TuTu owns a popular, local restaurant, featuring Hawaiian hamburgers and Harbor works at the restaurant in the drive-through which allows her the opportunity to practice ana-

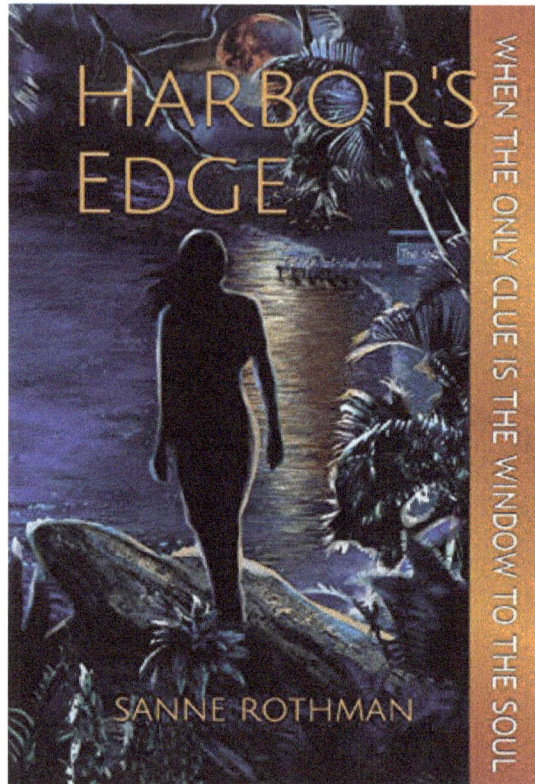

lyzing the faces of customers based on techniques from her father's FBI profiling manuals. She works on her skills at analyzing faces in the hopes of finding clues to her father's murderer and clues to her missing mother.

Overall a story filled with well-plotted twists and turns fueled by excitement and building tensions when children begin to turn up missing and Harbor thinks she may have a lead. Moreover, the story carries a mystery within a mystery as Harbor makes a friend at school, Keyne, with whom the sparks of first love begin to ignite, however, he seems to have an air of secrecy surrounding him as well.

Altogether, Harbor's Edge turned out to be both an imaginative and absorbing read that I thoroughly

enjoyed. I found myself instantly drawn into the beautifully set world of Harbor, shrouded in mystery, supernatural legacy, and artfully fueled with intriguing plot twists including, the unique inclusion of clues disbursed within each chapter. Additionally, I also enjoyed the likable characters within the story, especially that of Harbor. She's a relatable and intelligent character, easy to sympathize with and whose exciting journey to self-discovery was easy to follow. Absolutely, a worthwhile and noteworthy read that left me wanting more. I look forward to Book 2, Keyne, and The Wrath of The Mo'o. Overall, this would make a good choice for an end of summer read and I recommend it.

Source: EzineArticles

HOW TO MAKE A HYBRID WORK-FORCE SUCCESSFUL

With metrics for COVID-19 improving, many companies are starting to consider returning to work in person. But most employees and employers agree it won't look like it did before.

Indeed, research shows a large chunk of companies today are sizing their physical offices down, as more people work from home all the time or part of the week. And hybrid offices, arrangements where team members are in two or three days a week and work remotely the rest of the time, seem to be the wave of the future.

However, experts say that business owners and managers should not approach hybrid offices the same way they do completely remote set-ups.

"While there are very specific benefits to hybrid offices, they come with their own set of challenges," says Michele Havner, director of marketing at Eturi, the maker of Motiv, a recently-introduced app that small- and mid-sized business owners are using to improve productivity.

Motiv is a mobile dashboard that delivers important productivity metrics to CEOs, managers and leaders. The tool's reporting focuses on providing conference call activity and email summaries and integrates with Google Workspace and Microsoft 365, with many additional integrations and features slated for future release. Havner says that such tools function as a virtual corner office vantage point, helping to smooth out communication, collaboration and workflow issues created by hybrid arrangements and decentralized workspaces.

Equally important to communication is simply being mindful that hybrid offices can cause challenging dynamics among team members. Taking steps to address those issues preemptively can save headaches down the line. This includes making everyone accountable for meeting goals and deadlines. It might also mean offering the same perks to in-office and work-from-home staffers, while giving those who come into a centralized workspace the same level of flexibility remote work affords.

Easily adopted by small- and medium-sized businesses, which have been underserved by existing productivity solutions, Motiv is available through the iOS App Store and Google Play Store. To learn more, visit motivapp.com.

While hybrid offices can ultimately reduce costs and help keep employees healthy and safe, business owners will need to stay flexible and keep their workforce focused. Leveraging tools that facilitate hybrid work situations will be a key to success for companies as they move forward.

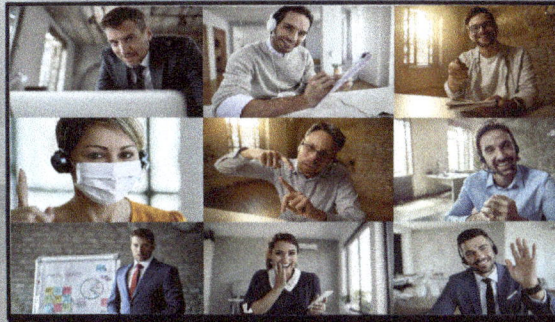

PHOTO BY DRAZEN ZIGIC / ISTOCK VIA GETTY IMAGES PLUS

INDEED, RESEARCH SHOWS A LARGE CHUNK OF COMPANIES TODAY ARE SIZING THEIR PHYSICAL OFFICES DOWN, AS MORE PEOPLE WORK FROM HOME ALL THE TIME OR PART OF THE WEEK.

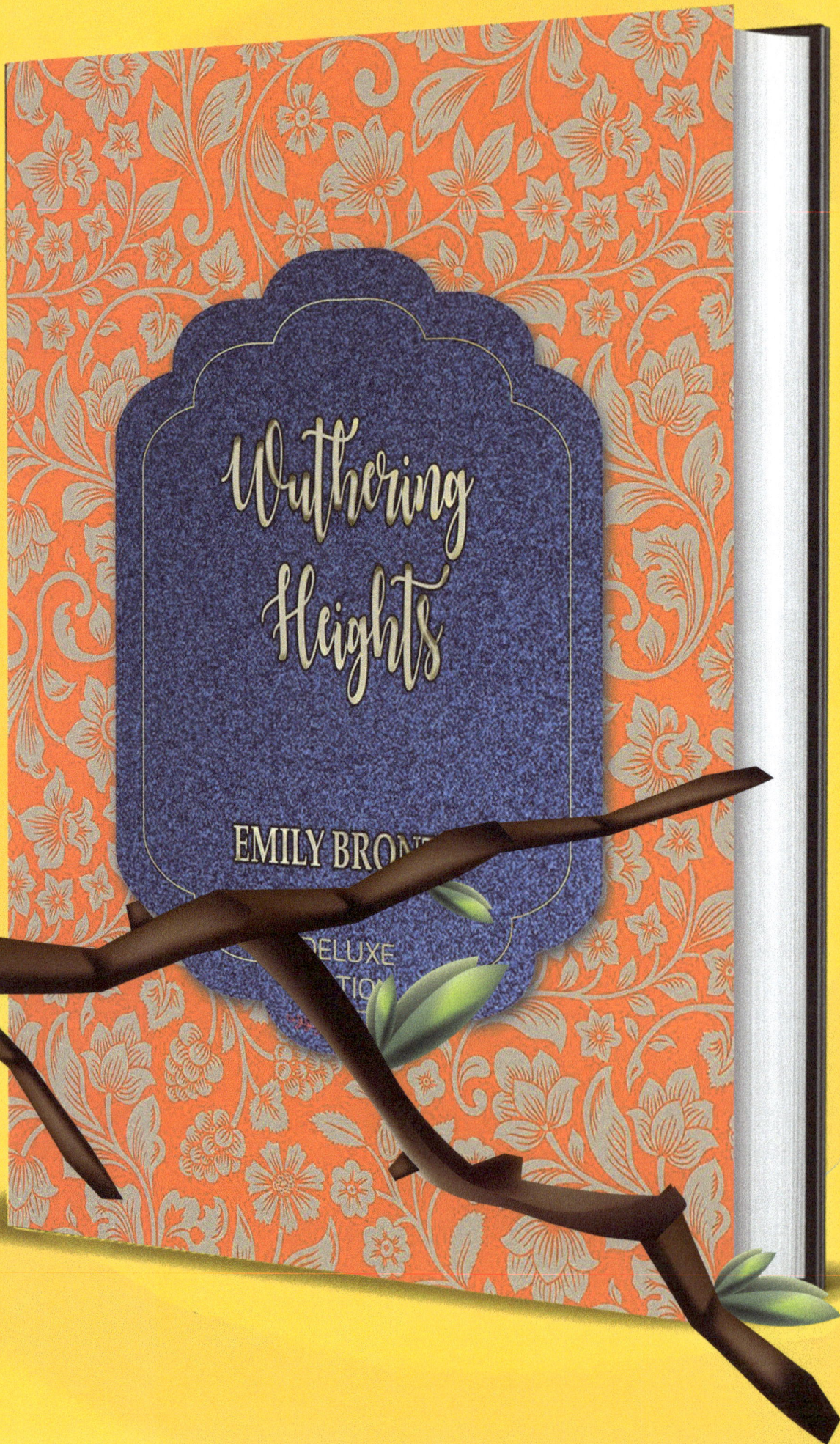

Wuthering Heights

EMILY BRONTË

DELUXE
EDITION

Deluxe Edition

Collected from the Guardiand's and
the Telegraph's "the 100 greatest novels of all time" list.

Preserved the original format whilst repairing
imperfections present in the aged copy.

See the complete list at
iboo.com

New

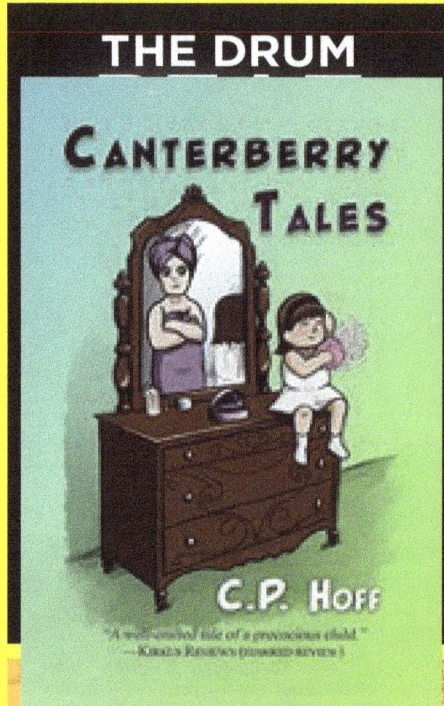

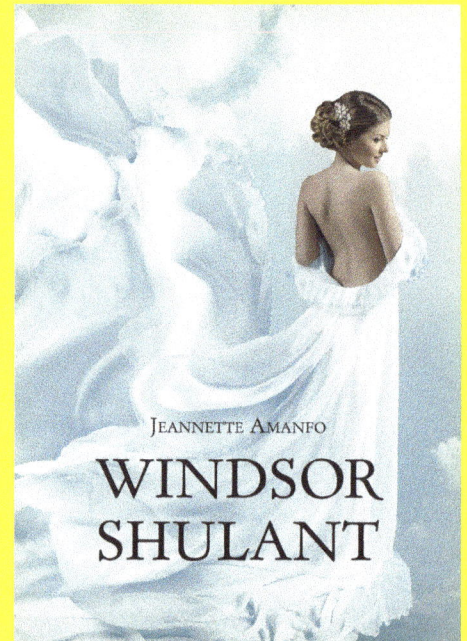

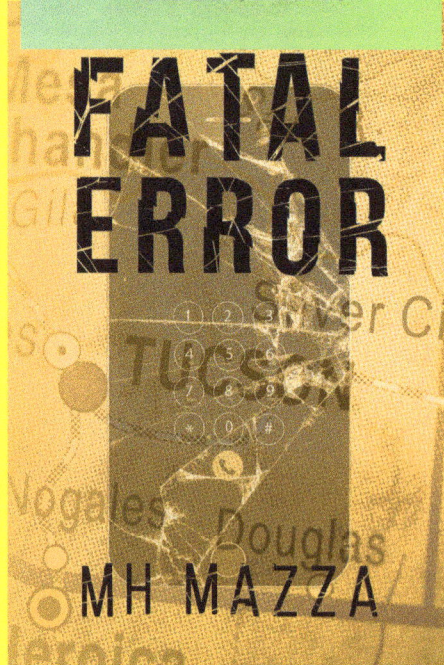

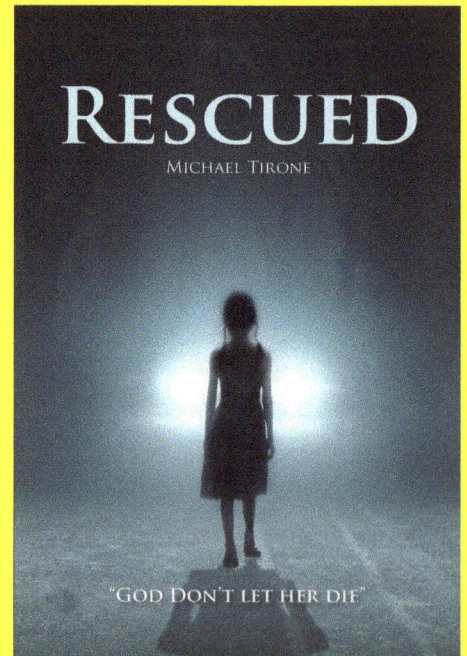

New

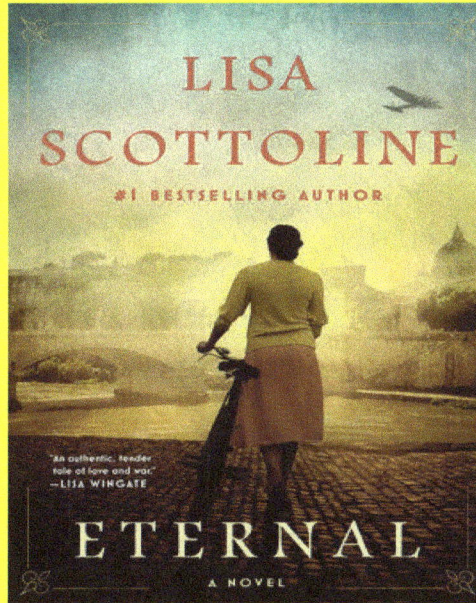

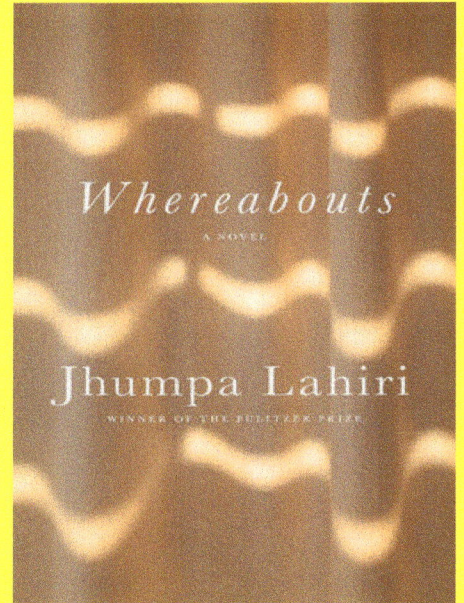

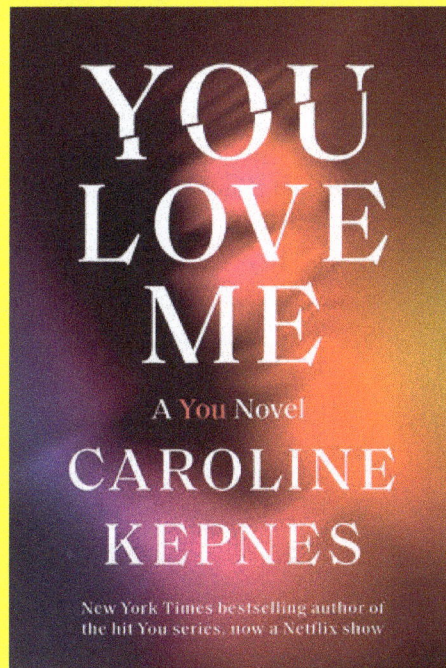

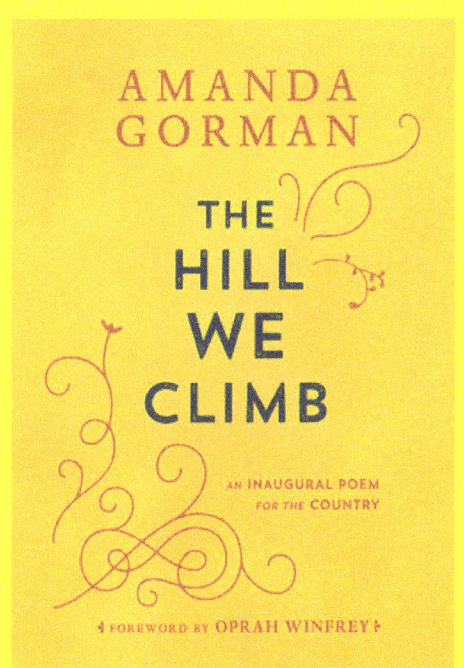

Genefitletics is a biotech venture that sequences & analyses human genes, and gut microbiome to translate complex biological data into technology driven, direct to customer actionable personalized dietary & lifestyle recommendations for intercepting & reversing chronic diseases, such as Irritable bowel Syndrome, Cardiovascular diseases, Depression, Anxiety, Acid Reflux, Crohn's, Parkinson's & Alzheimer's.
Hippocrates once said-
"Let the food be thy medicine & medicine be thy food".

When we talk of bacteria, what picture comes to our mind? A sneaky microorganism that does no good to us! But believe it or not, our gut houses trillions of bacteria! Ideally most of them are beneficial ones. Bringing a balance in gut bacteria- a balance between good & bad bacteria, where they belong to, and what functions they perform is the key to maintaining a healthy gut!

Why do we need to focus on gut health? Bacteria living in our body not only absorb nutrients, but also communicate with the brain, aid in the digestion process, improve our metabolism & regulate our immune health & hormone responses in our body. With so many beneficial functions being performed by these invisible friends living inside our gut, a healthy gut is the baseline for our overall holistic health.

With extensive research on gut health gaining popularity & results, and evidence showing that our gut bacteria influences every aspect of our health, taking care of these microbial army inside your body is the only way to be healthy & keep life threatening diseases such as Irritable bowel

GENEFITLETICS IS BRINGING THE NEXT WAVE OF DISRUPTION IN PRECISION NUTRITION

Syndrome, Cardiovascular diseases, Depression, Anxiety, Acid Reflux, Crohn's, Parkinson's & Alzheimer's at bay.

This has become more important with COVID-19 creating havoc globally!

Having the right kind of food that feeds beneficial bacteria in our gut is the only way to keep our gut in optimum balance. But how do we know what food is right for our gut?

Browsing for diet on Google, or resorting to supplements is not going to help. With a lot of fad diets such as ketosis, high protein or Atkins doing rounds; people have been made to believe that these diets are the best options available to improve their health.

However, these are generalized for a larger group of people. What works for your colleague may not work for you.

This has made people believe that having natural foods- green vegetables, fruits, whole grains having a lot of micronutrients will be healthy for them.

However it turns out that not all real foods- green vegetables or fruits will be healthy for you. Spinach may be good for your friend, but may be toxic for

The best way to learn what you should eat depends upon, which are the bacteria living in your gut, who are active & what they do inside your body. Without decoding your gut microbiome profile, it is virtually impossible to learn about- how those living in your gut are driving your overall health, be it metabolic, digestive or brain related.

you!

So what is THE solution? A personalized optimum diet unique for your body that feeds your gut bacteria & enables release of beneficial compounds, which helps your body grow and thrive.

WHO CAN TELL YOU WHAT IS BEST FOR YOUR BODY? WHAT SHOULD YOU EAT THAT CAN KEEP YOU AWAY FROM LIFE THREATENING DISEASES?

Solutions like Genefitletics can help you determine personalized food recommendations that will work for your body.

Our gut health is regulated by trillions of micro-organisms consisting of bacteria, algae, fungi, yeast & archaea. Genefitletics' UP THE GUT intelligence empowers you to bring healthy outcomes through insights from functional analysis of your gut microbiome.

THE BEST SOLUTION IS UNIQUE FOR YOUR BODY!

The best way to learn what you should eat depends upon, which are the bacteria living in your gut, who are active & what they do inside your body. Without decoding your gut microbiome profile, it is virtually impossible to learn about- how those living in your gut are driving your overall health, be it metabolic, digestive or brain related.

Therefore, you need a solution like Genefitletics that can enlighten you about the microbial ecosystem living inside your body, and what foods make them happy

enough to release beneficial compounds to help your body grow.

Genefitletics provides you personalised recommendations for the food you should eat more frequently, less frequently, minimise & avoid. Besides, the solution also tells you whether upon eating food, the gut bacteria in your colon releases toxins or breaks down the food into beneficial compounds such as short chain fatty acids.

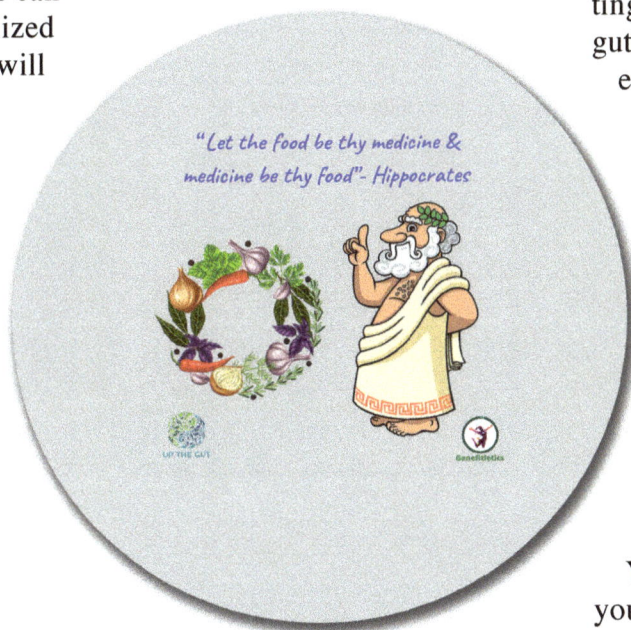

"Let the food be thy medicine & medicine be thy food"- Hippocrates

UP THE GUT

Genefitletics

SO HOW DO YOU GO ABOUT IT?

It's self explanatory! You need to sign up & pay for the solution. Genefitletics sends you a sample collection kit in which you take your stool sample. The kit is picked up by Genefitletics & processed in the lab. The results take about 4-6 weeks. During the entire process, you get regular emails & updates on the progress of sample processing & personalised diet recommendations upon completion of the sample anal-

ysis. Besides, during this period when the sample is in process, you also get a chance to participate in various quizzes & questionnaires which help you learn about your genetic predisposition to various foods such as milk, gluten and caffeine. This further helps you assess your overall risk of attracting lifestyle diseases.

WHAT IS THE USP?

Your entire 3 months program is divided into 3 phases- resetting your gut, optimising your gut & nourishing your gut. For each phase you get distinctive & unique food recommendations based on insights from your gut test evaluation. The best part is the raw & basic data from your gut analysis are converted into actionable personalised recommendations that you can depend & bank upon. All this, at a value deal of US $ 380 for a quarter.

You can also assess how well your gut is performing after you start following recommendations by doing a retest. Genefitletics offers retesting at a 10% discount.

When you start following a modified diet, you can start experiencing small positive changes such as reduced instances of bloating, less stress, high energy levels & better metabolism (to name some).

THE TAKEAWAY

Genefitletics uses an evidence based approach to give you a broad & detailed view about your gut ecosystem & community at a value deal with the objective of empowering you to improve your overall health without resorting to temporary reliefs.

New

New

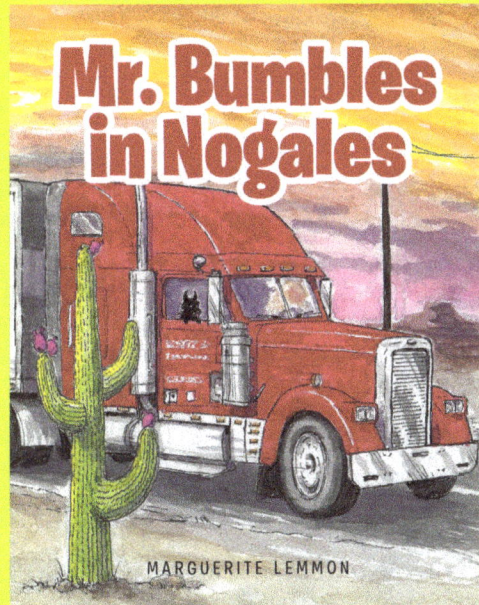
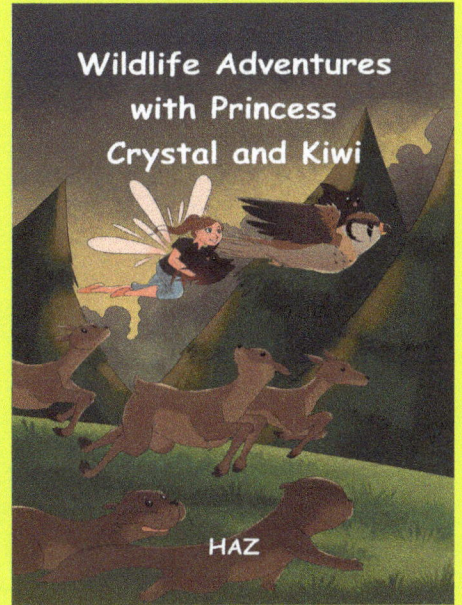
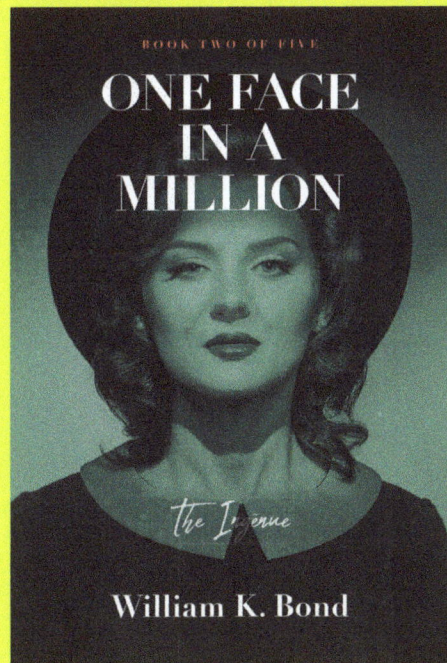
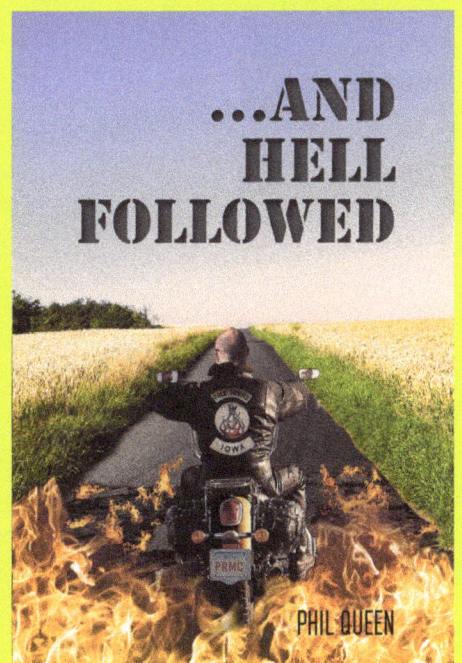

8
TIPS

Eight Tips to Prepare
FOR A VIRTUAL INTERVIEW

With these tips you will be well on your way to not only acing that interview, but job offers galore! Break a leg and most of all, be yourself, and let your personality shine!

BY RIAN DONATELLI

First and foremost, it is still a "real" interview, and should be treated as such. There is a person on the other end who will be making an executive decision about your qualifications for the job, so assume it's no different than if you met this individual in person.

Dress to impress! Even if they won't see your feet, dressing from head to toe in at least business casual attire is the first way to not only look professional when the camera goes live, but help you get into the right mindset. You'll be surprised how you will feel you can take on the world when you LOOK like you can!

Find a quiet and professional location for the interview. If you have a home office, this is perfect. If not, most libraries offer conference rooms free of charge, which you can reserve for yourself for the duration of the interview. There is nothing less professional than children, pets, or other household distractions infringing on your interview experience, and greatly affecting your appearance of professionalism. If you cannot get away from the home, set up at a dining room table or in a living room, and make sure everyone in the home knows you need some privacy for the allotted amount of time.

Try out the interview system in question before the interview. The day or night before, log on and familiarize yourself if it's a program you've never used. Even if it is something you use often, like Face-Time, double check that you have the contact info correct.

Pay close attention to the time zone the interviews are conducted in. This one is SO important. With the advent of virtual interviews, corporations have opened themselves up to a huge network of individuals all over the world, and while advantageous, also likely means they operate on a different time zone than yourself. No one wants to get off on a bad foot because you missed your interview or were late because you were unsure of the time zone. If it isn't clarified anywhere in a confirmation of any kind, reach out to your recruiter or interviewer, they will be happy to give you the information, and glad that you were proactive.

Try to use a laptop or desktop if at all possible, but if you have to use a Smartphone, set up a tripod system beforehand, so your hands can be free for the interview. You can even use a stack of books. What you don't want to do is hold the phone for the duration of the interview; this is a professional encounter, not a FaceTime chat with your grandma.

Like any interview, make sure you have studied up on the company and position you wish to hold. Google them. See if they have had any news lately. Did they recently merge with anyone? Or perhaps they made a branding change not long ago. In the very least, know the goods and/or services they offer, and be prepared to tell them how you could aid them in this niche if you were hired.

Prepare questions. Almost always the interviewer will ask you if you have any questions, and if they have answered all of them, its fine to tell them so. However, this is your chance to have their undivided attention, and ESPECIALLY if you are offered a job directly following. You will want to have compiled a list of anything you might have wanted to know, rather than bombarding the interviewer's inbox with emails less than 24 hours after they had time set aside to make themselves available just for you.

With these tips you will be well on your way to not only acing that interview, but job offers galore! Break a leg and most of all, be yourself, and let your personality shine!

Co-Author Colette Pfeiffer Talent Booking Experts & Connections Consulting and Marketing Solutions team.

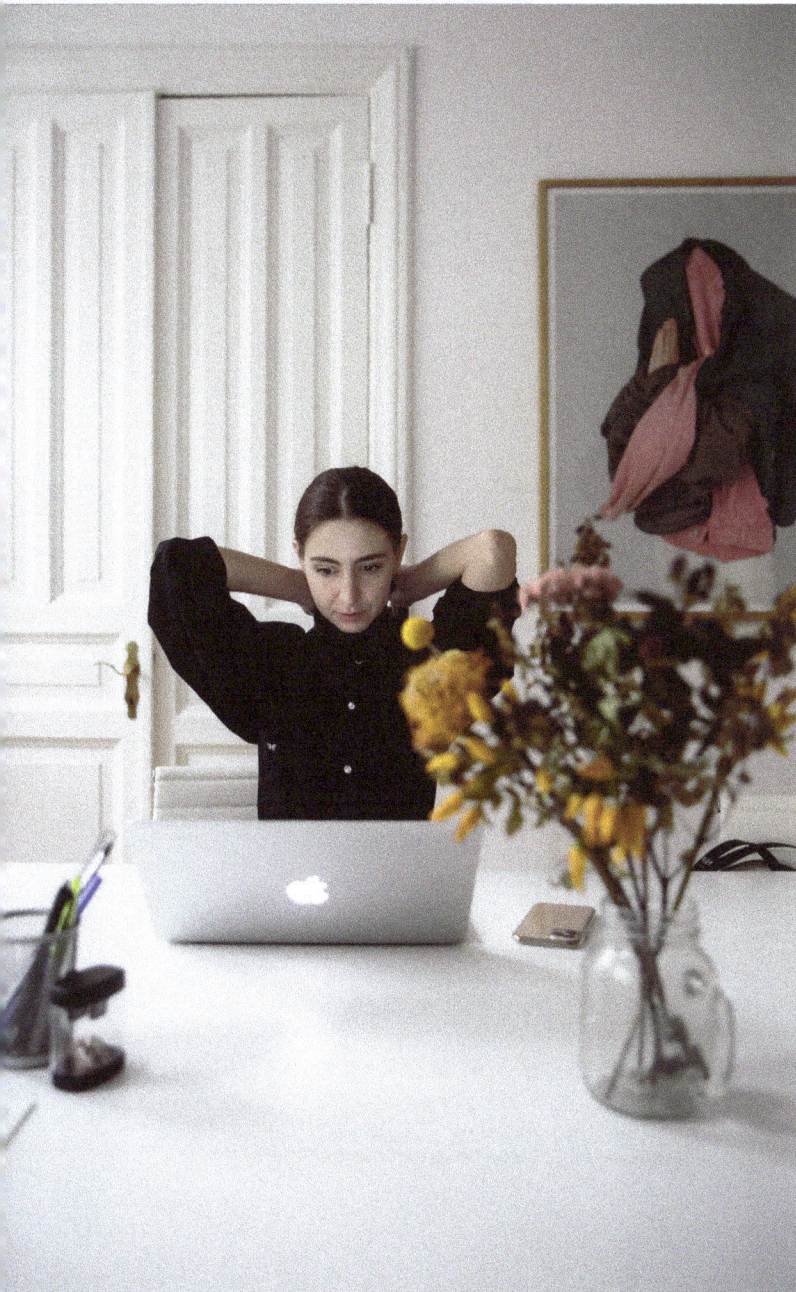

5 TIPS TO PUTTING A STOP TO BLOTCHY AND DISCOLORED SKIN

> **"** If left unaddressed, skin-discoloration conditions can interfere with people's ability to enjoy their everyday life – and, in some cases, can develop into more serious medical issues."

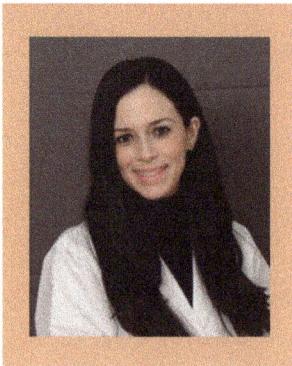

BY SHARON HOCHHAUSER, FNP-C

Heat, cold, sun, sweat, genes, hormones, stress…"Blotchy skin," notes Sharon Hochhauser, a board-certified family nurse practitioner specializing in dermatology with Advanced Dermatology PC, "can appear for many reasons. If left unaddressed, skin-discoloration conditions can interfere with people's ability to enjoy their everyday life – and, in some cases, can develop into more serious medical issues."

Our skin is our largest organ, with processes that require complex coordination of our body's systems. "If there is a misfire," explains Hochhauser, "we can end up with blotchy skin – reddened or discolored areas that can develop from

LIFESTYLE: BEAUTY

conditions such as eczema, rosacea, 'spider veins,' 'sun spots,' and melasma."

"Environmental triggers," Hochhauser continues, "can exacerbate underlying genetic conditions. Early identification of the causes of blotchy skin helps with management. And in cases where blotchy skin has become permanent, we have effective interventions to restore skin tone."

01

Keep your skin calm so blotches stay gone: "In particular," Hochhauser notes, "eczema and rosacea flares are susceptible to environmental triggers. The red patches of rosacea can develop gradually, with intermittent flushing that increases in duration and intensity. Early identification and reducing one's exposure to specific triggers, such as temperature extremes or spicy foods, can prevent more serious manifestations. Likewise, the red, itchy blotches of eczema can be exacerbated by environment, irritants, stress, and hormones. And both conditions require careful ongoing TLC, in particular gentle cleansing and regular moisturizing. Your skin care specialist can help you develop a management plan and choose products."

02

Zap! Laser spider-vein blotches away! "Over time," explains Hochhauser, "our veins may not work as efficiently, causing the appearance of red, web-like patches – medical name 'telangiectasia.' Especially if they appear on one's face, which can also occur with the repeated flushing of rosacea, broken blood vessels can be distressing. Laser treatments are an effective non-invasive we can remove the blotches of spider veins."

03

Get even with sunspots and melasma: "Both conditions," states Hochhauser, "result in darkened, blotchy skin due to overproduction of the skin pigment melanin. 'Sunspots' – solar lentigines – are the direct result of repeated sun exposure, whereas melasma, which typically affects women, can occur early on, with hormones playing a role. To remove and rejuvenate, we can use lasers to eliminate the underlying melanin-producing cells. Lasers can also restore unblemished skin, as can specialized exfoliation procedures such as microdermabrasion and chemical peels. Your skin-care specialist can also prescribe or recommend safe topical skin lighteners, which need to be chosen with care due to ongoing labeling issues that may hide the presence of dangerous ingredients like mercury."

04

Say 'YES!' to NO sun: "A common denominator of blotchy skin conditions," advises Hochhauser, "is the sun. Sun exposure can exacerbate symptoms, and, in some cases – for example, with solar lentigines – it is the cause. To help treatments last and prevent relapse, patients should be vigilant every day, all year: SPF 30 mineral sunscreen to block rays, plus protective clothing and seeking shade."

05

Not sure? See a doctor: "It's imperative," emphasizes Hochhauser, "to rule out dangerous conditions that require medical treatment, for example skin cancer. Your dermatologist's office can evaluate discolored skin to ensure that your condition is correctly identified and treated. With cases of rosacea and eczema, early identification is also important to jumpstart treatment that can slow progression. And with spider veins, it's important to check for circulatory issues."

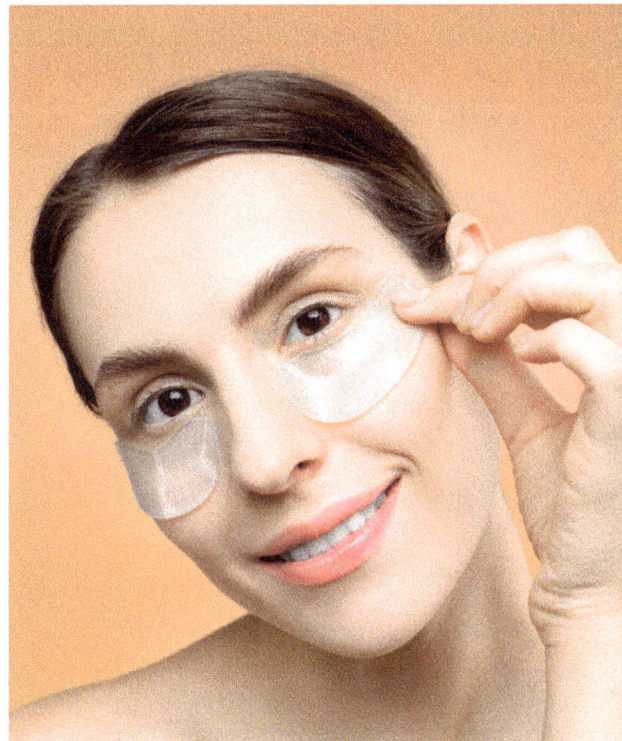

"Blotchy skin can show up for lots of reasons," concludes Hochhauser. "Fortunately, your dermatologist's office has interventions that can send it packing, too."
Sharon Hochhauser, MSN, RN, FNP-C, is a board-certified family nurse practitioner specializing in dermatology with Advanced Dermatology PC.

If you ask hardened scientists, they will say astrology can't work. On the other hand, believers will give the opposite opinion. And the truth is that both are right. Actually, it all depends upon the definition of "work". Basically, astrology refers to the belief that the stars and planets have an impact on a person's environment, personality, and mood based on when that person was born. Let's find out more.

You may have seen horoscopes published in newspapers. They are given by birth dates, and make predictions about people's lives and personalities. Besides, they give them advice based on the position of the astronomical bodies.

According to a survey done by the National Science Foundation, 41% respondents were of the opinion that astrology is kind of scientific.

The Position of Astronomical Bodies

The orientation and position of the sun in relation to Earth create seasons. We know that solar flares create electromagnetic disturbances on our planet. This process can cause blackouts and satellite disruptions. Besides, the moon position creates ocean tides. For instance, if you are a fisherman, the moon position can have an impact on your livelihood. On the other hand, the solar wind creates fascinating aura. And the biggest fact is that sunlight is the only biggest source of energy for us all.

Can Horoscopes make you Feel Better?

The short answer is, yes. The thing is that horoscopes can make you feel better. This is partly because of the placebo effect, which is a psychological effect. Basically, this effect happens when believing in a strange method makes you feel better.

Actually, it's the belief that makes you feel better, not the method. According to scientists, the placebo effect is proven. For instance, if you give tablets containing plain water to 10 patients and tell them the tablets can help them get better much sooner, many of the patients will get better. It's because of the placebo effect.

The new drug must perform much better than the placebo effect. In the experiment conducted by experts, the control group involved patients that received a placebo effect. Actually, this is the mechanism that makes astrology work for people.

You will find a lot of people who believe in astrology. They feel better when they follow the advice given in horoscopes. The same is true about a lot of pseudo-scientific treatments including homeopathy and crystal healing.

Actually, a new medicine shouldn't be proven to help patients feel better. There should be a proof that it works beyond the placebo effect. This is what we need to build a strong case.

If you stick to a scientifically proven treatment, you will have a belief that the treatment will work for you. For instance, you should go for a walk instead of reading horoscope in a newspaper. We know that exercise helps improve your mental and physical health.

Long story short, if you are into astrology, we suggest that you read this article again and review your understanding about horoscopy. Hopefully, you will find this article greatly helpful.

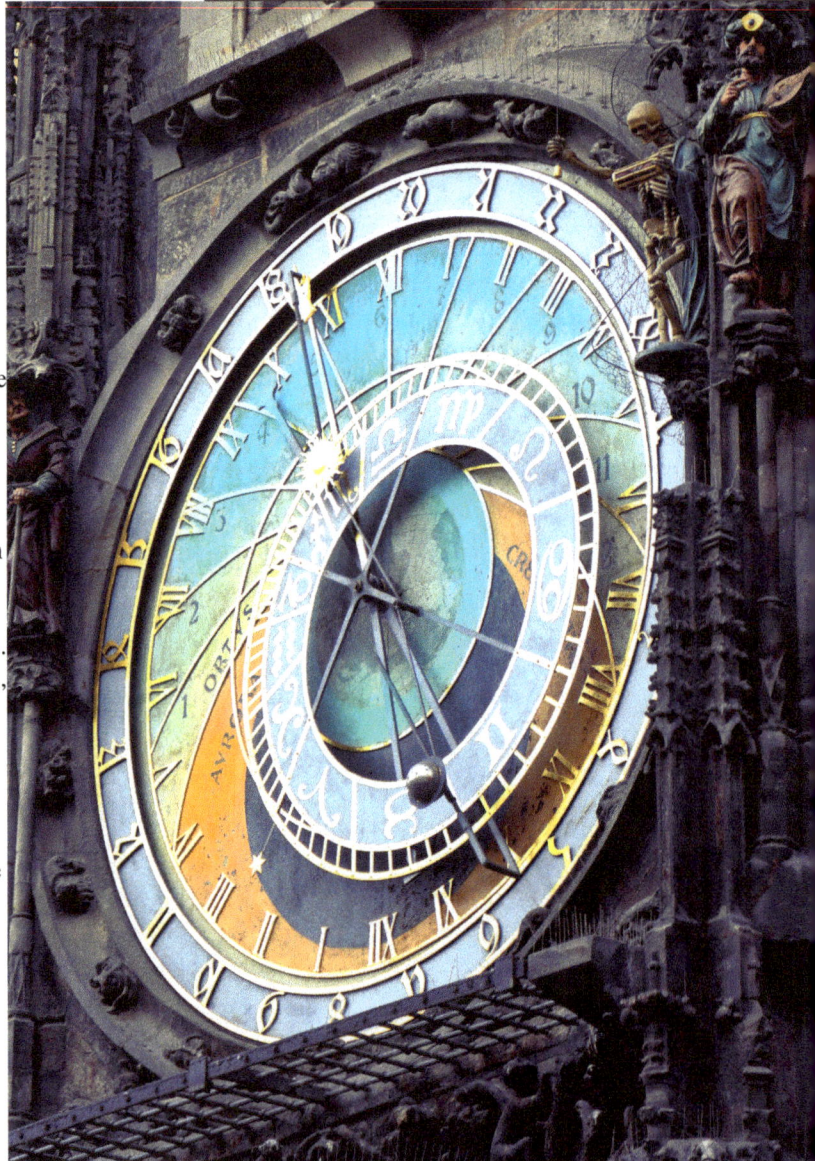

DOES ASTROLOGY REALLY WORK?

BY DHANUSUYA K

SOURCE: EzineArticles

BOOK REVIEW

1001 Movies You Must See Before You Die by Steven Jay Schneider

BY SANTHANAM NAGARAJAN

The book under review 1001 Movies You Must See Before You Die edited by Steven Jay Schneider gives you details of 1001 famous movies released between 1900 and 2016.

It is an elaborate work and a film lover's dream.

It chronicles the entire history of cinema spread over hundred years.

Choosing 1001 films from thousands of films is itself a research work and this was done by the author in a fantastic way.

How these films are chosen? First, from various best films, top hundred films, top ten movies lists 1300 films were selected. After going through the list again and again it was cut short to 1001 movies.

The films list is given alphabetically at the beginning of the book.

For example if you choose Tom Tykwer's Run Lola Run, a 1998 film, you will get all the details.

Run Lola Run is an interesting, unusual film making experiment that has humor, breathless excitement and tremendous energy all tightly packaged into an MTV generation movie by the fresh talent of its writer-director.

The film shows the twenty minute story of Lola in three different times each subtly different in a manner that delivers three different outcomes. A beautiful innovative film's full details are given in a fitting manner.

Like this you may read about one thousand and one best films and start viewing one by one before your death.

The Genre index given at the end of the book covers 22 subjects namely Action, Adventure, Animation, Avant-Garde, Comedy, Crime, Docu-drama, Documentary, Drama, Experimental, Family, Fantasy, Horror, Musical, Mystery, Noir, Romance, Sci-fi, Short, Thriller, War and Western.

The directors index gives you details about 596 famous director including Cecil B. Demille, Alfred Hitchcock, Steven Spielberg etc.

War films such The Bridge on the river Kwai

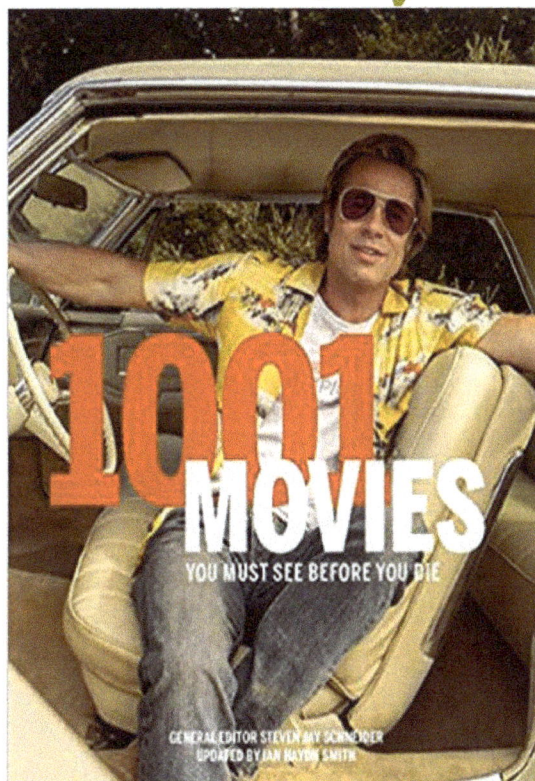

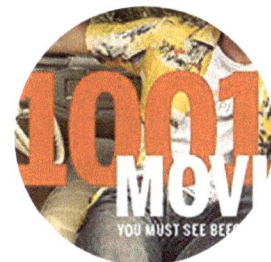

With over 1.75 million copies sold worldwide, this book is a must-have for all movie lovers, from casual movie-goers to film connoisseurs. This brand-new edition of 1001 Movies You Must See Before You Die covers more than a century of movie history. Selected and authored by a team of international film critics, every profile is packed with details, plot summaries and production notes, and little-known facts relating to the film's history. Each entry offers a fresh look at some the greatest films of all time.

Learn the complete history of filmmaking, from silent-era sensations such as D. W. Griffith's controversial The Birth of a Nation to recent Oscar winners. Discover little-known facts about Hollywood's most memorable musicals, greatest dramas, noteworthy documentaries, screwball comedies, classic westerns, action and adventure films, and more. Movie lovers of all stripes will thoroughly enjoy this must-have compilation.

(1957), The Great Escape (1963), Gone with the Wind (1939) needs to be specially mentioned here.

However we are not able to find the famous war films such The Guns of Navarone, Force Ten from Navarone etc.

Movies like The Italian Job are also not covered in this list.

Perhaps if we have to include all the films the title will become 10001 Movies you must see before you die!

Scientific Fiction films are also narrated elaborately.

The book is printed very neatly in art paper. Hundreds of illustration makes the reader very happy.

We may see and choose our favorite stars, Directors and we could make our own list based on our interest.

More than hundred years, the film field in one of the most entertaining one and we can't imagine a world without movies now. So we have to congratulate the General Editor Steven Jay Schneider for his painstaking work. He is a film critic, Scholar, and producer. He has written many books on the Cinematic arts.

Happy viewing of 1001 Movies!

Santhanam Nagarajan has written more than three thousand five hundred articles in Tamil and English. He has published 52 books so far. His articles on Mantras, Tantras, Scince and Hinduism are being read by thousands worldwide. He has appeared in more than 130 TV programmes.

Source: EzineArticles

www.ingramcontent.com/pod-product-compliance
Lightning Source LLC
Chambersburg PA
CBHW042355030426
42336CB00029B/3490